Beyond the Microscope: Nanotechnology's Impact on Our World

(Part 2)

Authored by

Shivang Dhoundiyal

&

Aftab Alam
Galgotias University, Greater Noida, India

Beyond the Microscope: Nanotechnology's Impact on Our World *(Part 2)*

Authors: Shivang Dhoundiyal & Aftab Alam

ISBN (Online): 979-8-89881-078-8

ISBN (Print): 979-8-89881-079-5

ISBN (Paperback): 979-8-89881-080-1

need for a court order if at any point you breach any terms of this License Agreement. In no event will any delay or failure by Bentham Science Publishers in enforcing your compliance with this License Agreement constitute a waiver of any of its rights.

3. You acknowledge that you have read this License Agreement, and agree to be bound by its terms and conditions. To the extent that any other terms and conditions presented on any website of Bentham Science Publishers conflict with, or are inconsistent with, the terms and conditions set out in this License Agreement, you acknowledge that the terms and conditions set out in this License Agreement shall prevail.

Bentham Science Publishers Pte. Ltd.
No. 9 Raffles Place
Office No. 26-01
Singapore 048619
Singapore
Email: subscriptions@benthamscience.net

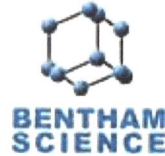

BENTHAM SCIENCE

CONTENTS

PREFACE

In Part 2 of this book, we shift our focus from theory to transformation. The following chapters showcase how nanotechnology is being applied to solve real-world problems across a variety of fields—from healing human bodies at the molecular level to protecting cultural heritage with invisible coatings.

We've written this section to illustrate what happens when cutting-edge science meets human needs. You'll read about personalized medical treatments, smart wearables that monitor your health, and nanomaterials that help preserve the planet. However, you'll also find discussions on the ethical boundaries and safety standards that must be upheld as this field continues to grow.

We aim to present nanotechnology as both a tool and a challenge—one that can do immense good when used wisely. We hope that these pages help you think critically, not only about what is possible, but also about what is right. As always, we thank you for joining us in exploring the infinitesimal wonders of nanoscience.

Shivang Dhoundiyal

&

Aftab Alam
Galgotias University, Greater Noida, India

CHAPTER 1

Nanotechnology in Agriculture and Food

Abstract: Nanotechnology offers transformative opportunities in agriculture and food, providing innovative solutions to enhance productivity, sustainability, and food safety. This chapter explores key applications of nanotechnology, including nanofertilizers for improved nutrient delivery, nanosensors for real-time monitoring of soil and plant health, and nano-pesticides for targeted pest control with reduced chemical use. These advancements contribute to more precise and efficient agricultural practices, boosting crop yields and minimizing environmental impact. In food preservation, nanocoatings extend shelf life and prevent contamination, while nanosensors ensure food safety by detecting pathogens and integrating into supply chain monitoring. Nanomaterials also enhance food processing, improving nutritional value, texture, and flavor. The chapter highlights smart delivery systems that control the release of nutrients and agrochemicals, alongside innovations in animal husbandry that improve health and productivity through advanced veterinary applications and feed supplements. It also discusses the environmental implications of nanotechnology, emphasizing the importance of assessing ecosystem impacts and developing regulatory frameworks to ensure safety. As nanotechnology continues to evolve, its potential to revolutionize agriculture and food systems is immense, promising a more sustainable, efficient, and resilient future in food production and security.

Keywords: Agriculture, Crops, Nanotechnology, Nanofertilizers, Nanosensors, Nanocoatings, Packaging.

INTRODUCTION

Nanotechnology, the science of manipulating matter at scales as small as one-billionth of a meter, is revolutionizing various sectors, including agriculture and food. This cutting-edge technology offers new tools and techniques that can significantly enhance food production and safety, contributing to more efficient, sustainable, and resilient agricultural systems [1]. The global demand for food is increasing due to population growth, climate change, and the depletion of natural resources, creating a pressing need for innovative solutions. Nanotechnology addresses these challenges by enabling precision agriculture, improving the efficiency of inputs like fertilizers and pesticides, and enhancing the quality and safety of food products [2]. As a result, it is becoming an indispensable component of modern agricultural practices and food systems. The applications of nanotechnology in agriculture are diverse and rapidly expanding, as mentioned in Table **1.1**. One of the most promising areas is precision farming, which leverages nanosensors and smart delivery systems to monitor and manage agricultural processes with unprecedented accuracy [3]. Nanosensors can detect soil moisture levels, nutrient deficiencies, and plant diseases early on, enabling timely interventions that improve crop health and yield. Nano-fertilizers and nano-pesticides are another significant application, designed to release nutrients and active compounds slowly and in a controlled manner, ensuring that plants receive the right amount at the right time. This not only enhances plant growth but also reduces the environmental impact of excess fertilizer and pesticide use, such as water contamination and soil degradation. In addition, nanotechnology is being used to develop nano-encapsulated agrochemicals, which protect active ingredients from degradation due to environmental factors, extending their efficacy. Nano-enabled delivery systems can also target specific plant tissues or pests, reducing the overall amount of chemicals needed and minimizing off-target effects [4]. Beyond crop management, nanotechnology is revolutionizing water purification and filtration systems, ensuring that irrigation water is free from contaminants that could harm crops or enter the food chain [5]. These advances contribute to more sustainable agricultural practices and improve the overall quality and safety of food products. Nanotechnology's importance in sustainable agriculture cannot be overstated. It offers numerous benefits that align with the principles of sustainability, including the efficient use of resources, reduced environmental impact, and enhanced food security. By enabling more precise application of inputs like water, fertilizers, and pesticides, nanotechnology reduces waste and mitigates the negative effects of overuse, such as soil degradation and water pollution. This is particularly crucial in regions facing water scarcity or where traditional farming practices have led to significant environmental degradation. Nanotechnology enhances the resilience of crops to environmental stressors like drought, salinity, and extreme temperatures, which are becoming more frequent and severe due to climate change. By improving plant health and reducing losses due to pests and diseases, nanotechnology helps to stabilize food production, even under challenging conditions. This is vital for ensuring food security, especially in developing regions where agricultural productivity is closely linked to livelihoods and economic stability. Another key benefit of nanotechnology is its potential to reduce post-harvest losses through advanced packaging and preservation techniques. Nano-enabled packaging materials can detect spoilage, extend shelf life, and even release preservatives in a controlled manner, ensuring that food remains fresh from farm to table [6]. This helps reduce food waste, a significant issue in the global food supply chain, and ensures that more of the food produced reaches consumers.

Table 1.1. Role of nanotechnology in agriculture and food.

Area	Application	Benefits	References
Crop Yield Enhancement	Nanofertilizers	Improved nutrient delivery, enhanced crop yield, reduced environmental impact.	[7]
-	Nanosensors for Crop Monitoring	Real-time soil and plant health monitoring, precision agriculture.	[8]
-	Nano-pesticides	Targeted pest control, reduced chemical use, and minimized environmental impact.	[9]
Food Preservation	Nanocoatings for Food Packaging	Extending shelf life, preventing contamination, and maintaining food quality.	[10]
-	Nanosensors for Food Safety	Detection of pathogens and contaminants, integration into supply chain monitoring.	[11]
-	Nanomaterials in Food Processing	Enhancing food quality, improving nutritional value, and innovating texture and flavor.	[12]
Animal Husbandry	Smart Delivery Systems	Controlled release of nutrients and agrochemicals, and increased efficiency and productivity.	[13]
-	Nanotechnology in Veterinary Medicine and Feed Supplements	Improved animal health, enhanced productivity, and targeted delivery of veterinary drugs and supplements.	[14]
Environmental and Safety	Regulatory Frameworks and Safety Standards	Ensuring environmental and human safety, and guiding the responsible use of nanotechnology.	[15]

ENHANCING CROP YIELD AND PROTECTION

Nano Fertilizers

Nanofertilizers represent a groundbreaking advancement in agricultural technology, designed to improve the efficiency and effectiveness of nutrient delivery to plants. Traditional fertilizers often suffer from issues such as nutrient leaching, volatilization, and inefficient uptake by plants, leading to significant wastage and environmental pollution [16]. Nanofertilizers, on the other hand, utilize nanoscale materials to encapsulate or coat nutrients, allowing for more precise and controlled release [17]. This targeted approach ensures that nutrients are delivered directly to the plant roots, enhancing absorption and reducing the amount of fertilizer needed. As a result, nanofertilizers not only improve the nutritional content available to crops but also minimize the negative environmental impacts associated with excessive fertilizer use [18]. The core innovation behind nanofertilizers lies in their advanced nutrient delivery systems. These systems are engineered to release nutrients in a slow and sustained manner, matching the specific growth stages and nutrient demands of crops. For instance, nanomaterials can be designed to respond to environmental triggers such as soil pH, moisture levels, or root exudates, releasing nutrients only when the plants need them [19]. This level of precision not only maximizes nutrient uptake by plants but also reduces the risk of nutrient runoff into water bodies, which can cause eutrophication and other ecological problems. Additionally, nanofertilizers can be formulated to include multiple nutrients in a single application, addressing the specific needs of crops more comprehensively than conventional fertilizers. This multi-nutrient approach not only boosts plant growth and yield but also enhances soil health by maintaining a balanced nutrient profile. The efficacy of nanofertilizers has been demonstrated in various case studies, showcasing their potential to significantly increase crop yields. In one study, the application of nano-encapsulated nitrogen fertilizers to wheat crops resulted in a 20-30% increase in grain yield compared to traditional fertilizers [20]. The slow and controlled release of nitrogen reduced losses due to volatilization and leaching, ensuring that more of the applied nitrogen was available to the plants throughout the growing season. Similarly, in rice cultivation, the use of nanofertilizers containing essential micronutrients such as zinc and iron led to improved plant health, increased resistance to diseases, and higher grain production. Another notable example is the application of nano-hydroxyapatite as a phosphate fertilizer, which has been shown to enhance phosphorus availability in the soil, leading to better root development and higher crop yields in maize.

Nanosensors for Crop Monitoring

Nanosensors are a cutting-edge innovation in agricultural technology, designed to monitor crop health and soil conditions with high precision and in real-time. These tiny devices, often no larger than a few nanometers, are embedded with the capability to detect and measure a wide range of environmental parameters, including soil moisture, nutrient levels, pH, temperature, and the presence of pests or diseases [21]. The use of nanosensors in agriculture enables farmers to gather detailed, accurate data on their crops and soil conditions, allowing for timely and informed decision-making. This technology is integral to the advancement of precision agriculture, where the goal is to optimize the use of resources, enhance crop yields, and reduce environmental impacts through targeted interventions. One of the most significant advantages of nanosensors is their ability to provide real-time monitoring of soil and plant health. Traditional methods of soil and crop analysis often involve manual sampling and laboratory testing, which can be time-consuming, labor-intensive, and subject to delays. In contrast, nanosensors can be deployed directly in the field, continuously collecting data and transmitting it to farmers *via* wireless networks [22]. This constant stream of information allows for immediate detection of issues such as nutrient deficiencies, water stress, or disease onset, enabling farmers to take corrective actions before these problems escalate. For example, nanosensors can detect early signs of drought stress by monitoring soil moisture levels and signaling when irrigation is needed, thus preventing crop damage and optimizing water use. Similarly, by tracking nutrient levels, these sensors can help ensure that plants receive the right amount of fertilizers at the right time, enhancing nutrient uptake and reducing wastage. Nanosensors are at the forefront of precision agriculture, a farming management concept that uses technology to observe, measure, and respond to field variability in crops. Precision agriculture aims to optimize field-level management regarding crop farming by assessing the needs of individual plants or specific areas within a field, rather than applying a uniform treatment to the entire field [23]. Nanosensors play a crucial role in this approach by providing detailed, localized data that guides precise applications of water, fertilizers, and pesticides. For instance, in large-scale farming, nanosensors can map out areas of a field that require more attention, such as zones with poor soil quality or higher pest activity. This enables farmers to apply resources more efficiently, targeting only the areas that need treatment, thereby reducing input costs and minimizing environmental impacts. The role of nanosensors with GPS and drone technologies allows for automated monitoring and intervention, further enhancing the efficiency and effectiveness of farm management practices [24]. The use of nanosensors in precision agriculture also supports sustainable farming practices. By reducing the overuse of fertilizers and pesticides, these sensors help lower the risk of soil degradation and water contamination, which are common issues in conventional farming methods. The ability to monitor crops and soil in real-time contributes to more resilient agricultural systems, capable of adapting to changing environmental conditions and mitigating the effects of climate change.

Nano-pesticides

Nano-pesticides represent a transformative advancement in pest management, utilizing nanotechnology to enhance the effectiveness, precision, and safety of pesticide applications. Traditional pesticides, while effective, often face challenges such as rapid degradation, inefficient delivery, and non-specific targeting, which can lead to excessive chemical use, environmental contamination, and harm to non-target organisms. Nano-pesticides address these issues by incorporating active ingredients into nanoscale carriers or encapsulating them within nanomaterials, which can be engineered to release the pesticide in a controlled and sustained manner [25]. This innovative approach not only improves the stability and bioavailability of the active ingredients but also allows for targeted pest control, minimizing the overall amount of chemicals required and reducing the environmental footprint of pest management practices. One of the key advantages of nano-pesticides is their ability to deliver targeted pest control. By designing nanoparticles that can recognize and bind to specific pest organisms or plant tissues, nano-pesticides can ensure that the active ingredients are released precisely where they are needed, and in the right amounts. This targeted delivery minimizes off-target effects, reducing the impact on beneficial insects, soil microorganisms, and surrounding vegetation. Additionally, the controlled release mechanisms of nano-pesticides mean that the active compounds are gradually released over time, maintaining effective pest control for longer periods and reducing the need for frequent reapplication [26]. This results in significant reductions in the overall quantity of pesticides used, lowering costs for farmers and decreasing the risk of pesticide resistance developing in pest populations. By using nano-pesticides, farmers can achieve more effective pest management with less environmental disruptions, contributing to more sustainable agricultural practices. While nano-pesticides offer numerous benefits, their environmental impact and safety considerations are critical aspects that must be carefully managed [27]. The use of nanomaterials in agriculture introduces new variables in terms of toxicity, bioaccumulation, and the potential for unintended ecological consequences. It is essential to ensure that the nanomaterials used in these pesticides do not persist in the environment or accumulate in non-target organisms, where they could cause harm. Rigorous testing and regulation are necessary to assess the long-term effects of nano-pesticides on soil health, water quality, and biodiversity. Additionally, the development of biodegradable or environmentally benign nanomaterials is a priority to minimize any potential negative impacts. Despite these concerns, nano-pesticides hold the promise of reducing the overall environmental burden associated with conventional pesticide use. By lowering the amount of chemical inputs needed and enhancing their efficiency, nano-pesticides can help reduce the contamination of water bodies, soil degradation, and harm to non-target species [28]. Furthermore, by enabling more precise pest control, they can contribute to the reduction of pesticide residues in food products, enhancing food safety for consumers. The continued research and development of nano-pesticides, coupled with robust safety assessments and regulatory frameworks, will be crucial in ensuring that their adoption in agriculture leads to positive outcomes for both food production and environmental sustainability.

FOOD PRESERVATION AND SAFETY

Nanocoatings for Food Packaging

Nanocoatings for food packaging are an innovative application of nanotechnology that plays a crucial role in extending the shelf life of food products and preventing contamination. These ultra-thin, nanoscale layers are applied to packaging materials to create protective barriers that are highly effective against moisture, gases, and microbial contaminants. Traditional food packaging often struggles to maintain the freshness of perishable items, leading to spoilage and significant food waste [29]. Nanocoatings address these challenges by offering enhanced barrier properties, such as improved resistance to oxygen and water vapor transmission, which are critical factors in preserving the quality and safety of food. Nanocoatings can be designed with antimicrobial properties, actively inhibiting the growth of bacteria, fungi, and other pathogens on the food surface, thereby reducing the risk of foodborne illnesses [30]. This innovative approach not only improves the longevity of food products but also contributes to food safety and reduces the reliance on chemical preservatives. The primary function of nanocoatings in food packaging is to extend the shelf-life of food products by creating a more effective barrier against external factors that contribute to spoilage [31]. By controlling the exchange of gases like oxygen and carbon dioxide, as well as moisture, nanocoatings help maintain the optimal internal environment of the packaging, slowing down the degradation processes of food items. For example, fruits and vegetables often release ethylene gas as they ripen, which can accelerate spoilage if not properly managed [32]. Nanocoatings can incorporate ethylene scavengers that capture and neutralize this gas, thereby extending the freshness of produce. Additionally, nanocoatings can be infused with antimicrobial agents, which actively protect food from microbial contamination throughout the supply chain. This is particularly important for perishable items such as dairy products, meats, and seafood, where contamination risks are high. By preventing microbial growth, nanocoatings help ensure that food remains safe to consume, even under fluctuating storage conditions. Nanocoatings have diverse applications in both perishable and processed foods, making them an essential technology in modern food packaging. For perishable foods, such as fresh fruits, vegetables, meats, and dairy products, nanocoatings provide a protective layer that helps to retain moisture, prevent oxidation, and inhibit microbial activity [33]. This not only preserves the taste, texture, and nutritional value of the food but also reduces food waste by extending the time these products remain fresh and safe to eat. In processed foods, nanocoatings can be used to improve the packaging of items like snacks, baked goods, and ready-to-eat meals by enhancing barrier properties that protect against environmental factors like humidity and oxygen, which can cause staleness or rancidity. The versatility of nanocoatings allows for their application in various packaging materials, including plastics, paper, and even biodegradable options. In the packaging of processed foods, nanocoatings can be used to create active packaging that not only protects the food but also interacts with it to release preservatives or absorb unwanted substances, such as excess moisture or odors

[34]. This adaptive functionality is particularly beneficial for maintaining the quality of processed foods during long storage or transportation periods.

Nanosensors for Food Safety

Nanosensors are emerging as a powerful tool in food safety, offering advanced capabilities for the rapid and accurate detection of pathogens and contaminants in food products. These nanoscale sensors are designed to detect minute traces of harmful substances, such as bacteria, viruses, toxins, heavy metals, and chemical residues, that can compromise food safety and pose significant health risks to consumers [35]. Traditional methods of detecting contaminants in food often involve time-consuming laboratory tests, which may delay the identification of foodborne hazards and lead to widespread outbreaks before action can be taken. Nanosensors, on the other hand, can provide real-time, on-site detection, enabling immediate responses to potential threats. By incorporating highly sensitive nanomaterials, such as nanoparticles, nanotubes, and nanowires, these sensors can identify contaminants at extremely low concentrations, offering a level of precision and speed that surpasses conventional testing methods [36]. This capability is crucial for ensuring the safety of food products from the point of production through to consumption. The detection of pathogens and contaminants is a critical application of nanosensors in food safety. These nanosensors can be engineered to recognize specific molecular signatures associated with harmful microbes or chemical substances. For example, nanosensors can be functionalized with antibodies, DNA sequences, or other biomolecules that selectively bind to the surface proteins or genetic material of pathogens like *E. coli, Salmonella*, or *Listeria* [37]. Once the target pathogen is detected, the nanosensor generates a detectable signal, such as a change in color, fluorescence, or electrical current, indicating the presence of contamination. This rapid detection capability allows for timely intervention, such as the removal of contaminated products from the supply chain, before they reach consumers. Additionally, nanosensors can be used to monitor for allergens, pesticide residues, and other harmful chemicals, ensuring that food products meet safety standards and are free from substances that could trigger adverse health effects. Nanosensors in supply chain monitoring systems represent a significant advancement in ensuring food safety from farm to table. The food supply chain is complex and involves multiple stages, including production, processing, packaging, transportation, and retail. At each stage, there is potential for contamination to occur, making continuous monitoring essential [38]. Nanosensors can be embedded in packaging materials, storage environments, and transport containers to provide real-time data on the condition of food products as they move through the supply chain. For instance, nanosensors can monitor temperature, humidity, and the presence of spoilage indicators, providing early warnings of compromised conditions that could lead to contamination or spoilage. This real-time data can be transmitted to central monitoring systems, allowing for immediate corrective actions, such as adjusting storage conditions, rerouting shipments, or recalling products before they reach consumers. The use of nanosensors in supply chain monitoring enhances traceability and transparency, key components of modern food safety systems [39]. By continuously tracking the condition of food products and detecting any signs of contamination, nanosensors help build trust between producers, retailers, and consumers. They also provide valuable data for improving supply chain management practices, reducing food waste, and ensuring compliance with food safety regulations. As the technology evolves, the potential to use nanosensors with other smart technologies, such as blockchain and the Internet of Things (IoT), could further enhance the accuracy, reliability, and efficiency of food safety monitoring across global supply chains [40].

Nanomaterials in Food Processing

Nanomaterials, which operate at the nanoscale, have unique properties that allow them to interact with food components in ways that are not possible with conventional ingredients or additives. In food processing, nanomaterials can be used to improve the stability and bioavailability of nutrients, protect sensitive ingredients during processing, and create novel textures and flavors that enhance the overall consumer experience. The use of nanotechnology in this domain is paving the way for the development of healthier, more enjoyable, and longer-lasting food products, addressing consumer demands for both quality and nutrition [41]. Nanomaterials play a critical role in enhancing the quality and nutritional value of food products. One of the key applications is the encapsulation of vitamins, minerals, and other bioactive compounds in nanocarriers, which protects these nutrients from degradation during processing and storage. This ensures that the nutrients remain potent until the point of consumption, significantly increasing their effectiveness. For instance, omega-3 fatty acids, which are prone to oxidation, can be encapsulated in nanoemulsions to prevent spoilage and preserve their health benefits in functional foods [42]. Additionally, nanomaterials can be designed to improve the absorption of nutrients in the body. Nano-sized particles have a larger surface area and can more easily penetrate biological barriers, making nutrients more bioavailable. This is particularly important for enhancing the delivery of essential nutrients like iron, calcium, and vitamins, which can be challenging to absorb in sufficient quantities from conventional food sources. Beyond improving nutritional content, nanomaterials are also revolutionizing the way food is experienced in terms of texture and flavor. In food processing, nanomaterials can be used to create novel textures that are otherwise difficult to achieve [43]. For example, nanoparticles can be used to stabilize emulsions, resulting in creamy textures in low-fat products that mimic the mouthfeel of full-fat versions. This allows food manufacturers to produce healthier alternatives without compromising on sensory appeal. Additionally, nanomaterials can be engineered to control the release of flavors, providing a more intense and prolonged taste experience. For example, nanocapsules containing flavor compounds can be designed to break down at specific points during chewing or digestion, releasing flavors in stages and enhancing the overall taste experience [44]. They also enable the modification of food structures at a molecular level, allowing for the creation of innovative food products with unique properties. For instance, aerogels and nanofoams can be incorporated into foods to create light, airy textures that add novelty and appeal to traditional products. The ability to manipulate food at the nanoscale also opens up possibilities for developing customized flavors and textures tailored to individual preferences or dietary needs, offering a more personalized eating experience.

INNOVATIONS IN AGRI-NANOTECH

Smart delivery systems utilize nanomaterials to encapsulate or bind active ingredients, such as fertilizers, pesticides, herbicides, or growth regulators, and release them in a controlled, targeted manner over time. Traditional agricultural practices often involve the application of large quantities of chemicals, much of which can be lost due to volatilization, leaching, or degradation before they benefit the crops [45]. Smart delivery systems address these inefficiencies by ensuring that active ingredients are delivered directly to the plants or soil, precisely when and where they are needed, thereby maximizing their efficacy while minimizing environmental impact and reducing costs. The core feature of smart delivery systems is their ability to control the release of nutrients and agrochemicals, tailored to the specific needs of crops throughout their growth cycle. This is achieved through the use of nanocarriers, such as liposomes, polymeric nanoparticles, and nanoclays, which can be engineered to respond to various environmental triggers like pH, temperature, or moisture levels. For example, a smart delivery system might release nutrients in response to the moisture level in the soil, ensuring that plants receive nourishment during critical growth phases or in response to drought conditions [46]. Similarly, pesticides encapsulated in nanocarriers can be released gradually, providing prolonged protection against pests and reducing the frequency of applications. This precision in timing and location not only enhances the effectiveness of the agrochemicals but also significantly reduces the risk of runoff and contamination of water bodies, soil degradation, and harm to non-target organisms. The practical benefits of smart delivery systems have been demonstrated in various field applications, showcasing their potential to revolutionize modern agriculture. One notable case study involved the use of nano-encapsulated fertilizers in rice cultivation. In this study, the smart delivery system enabled a slow and sustained release of nitrogen, which significantly increased nitrogen use efficiency and resulted in a 20-30% improvement in crop yield compared to conventional fertilizers [47]. Another example is the use of smart delivery systems for herbicides in maize fields, where the controlled release of herbicides reduced weed growth while minimizing the impact on soil health and non-target plant species [48]. In a similar vein, a study on tomato plants demonstrated that using nanocarrier-based pesticides resulted in better pest control and higher fruit yield, with fewer pesticide applications required throughout the growing season. These case studies highlight the potential of smart delivery systems to enhance agricultural productivity, reduce input costs, and promote sustainable farming practices. By improving the efficiency and effectiveness of nutrient and agrochemical applications, these systems contribute to the overall goal of precision agriculture, where inputs are used more judiciously, and environmental impacts are minimized, as depicted in Fig. (**1.1**). As smart delivery technologies continue to evolve, they hold the promise of further innovations in agriculture, helping to meet the growing global demand for food in a more sustainable and resource-efficient manner.

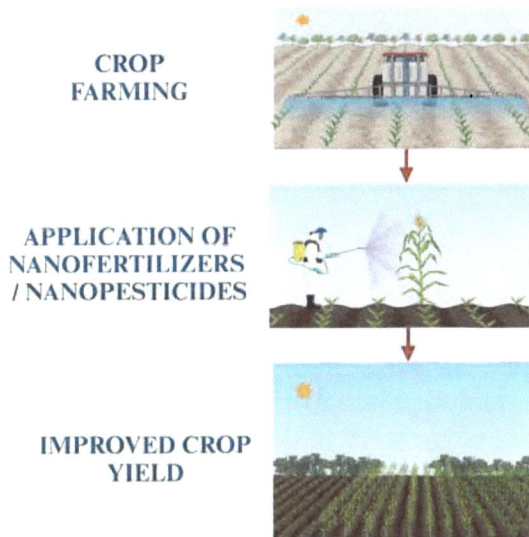

CROP FARMING

APPLICATION OF NANOFERTILIZERS / NANOPESTICIDES

IMPROVED CROP YIELD

Fig. (1.1). Role of nanofertilizers/nano pesticides in improving crop yield.

Nanotechnology in Animal Husbandry

Nanotechnology is increasingly being applied in animal husbandry to improve animal health, enhance productivity, and advance veterinary medicine. Their role in this field offers innovative solutions to long-standing challenges, such as disease management, nutrient absorption, and the efficient delivery of veterinary drugs. By utilizing nanoscale materials and technologies, animal husbandry practices can become more precise, efficient, and sustainable. Nanotechnology can help optimize the health and well-being of livestock, leading to higher productivity and better-quality animal products, while also addressing concerns about antibiotic resistance, animal welfare, and environmental impact. One of the most significant contributions of nanotechnology to animal husbandry is the enhancement of animal health and productivity [49]. Nanomaterials can be used to improve the delivery of essential nutrients and supplements, ensuring that animals receive the right amounts of vitamins, minerals, and other critical nutrients. For example, nano-encapsulated feed additives can enhance the bioavailability of nutrients, leading to better growth rates, improved immune function, and overall better health outcomes for livestock. This is particularly important in intensive farming systems, where ensuring optimal nutrition is key to maintaining animal health and maximizing production efficiency. Nanotechnology enables the development of advanced diagnostic tools, such as nanosensors and nanobiosensors, which can detect diseases and health issues at an early stage, allowing for timely intervention and reducing the spread of infections [50]. By ensuring that animals remain healthy and productive, nanotechnology helps to increase the yield and quality of products such as meat, milk, and eggs, contributing to the overall efficiency and profitability of animal husbandry operations. Nanotechnology is also revolutionizing veterinary medicine and the development of feed supplements. In veterinary medicine, nanotechnology is being used to create more effective and targeted drug delivery systems. These systems can deliver medications directly to the site of infection or inflammation, reducing the required dosage and minimizing side effects. For example, nanoparticles can be used to encapsulate antibiotics, antiparasitics, or anti-inflammatory drugs, ensuring that these medications are released in a controlled manner and at the optimal therapeutic concentration [51]. This targeted approach not only improves the efficacy of treatments but also helps to mitigate the growing concern of antibiotic resistance by reducing the need for broad-spectrum antibiotics. In feed supplements, nanotechnology offers solutions for enhancing the nutritional content and stability of feed additives. Nano-encapsulation protects sensitive ingredients, such as probiotics, enzymes, and vitamins, from degradation during storage and digestion, ensuring that these beneficial compounds are effectively delivered to the animals. This leads to improved digestion, nutrient absorption, and overall growth performance. For instance, the use of nano-minerals, such as nano-selenium or nano-zinc, in feed supplements has been shown to enhance immune response, reproductive performance, and stress resistance in livestock, compared to their conventional counterparts [52]. Moreover, the application of nanotechnology in animal husbandry extends to the development of vaccines. Nano-vaccines are being explored for their potential to induce stronger and more specific immune responses, with fewer doses and better protection against diseases. These vaccines can be engineered to mimic the natural infection process, stimulating the immune system more effectively and offering long-lasting immunity. This advancement is particularly valuable in controlling infectious diseases that can devastate livestock populations and pose risks to food security.

Environmental Implications and Regulatory Considerations

As nanotechnology rapidly advances across various sectors, including agriculture, food production, and animal husbandry, understanding its environmental implications and ensuring robust regulatory oversight are critical, as depicted in Fig. (**1.2**). The unique properties of nanomaterials—such as their small size, high reactivity, and potential to interact with biological systems in unprecedented ways—mean they could have significant impacts on ecosystems and human health [53]. Assessing these impacts involves understanding how nanomaterials behave in the environment, their potential for bioaccumulation, and their effects on soil, water, air, and living organisms. At the same time, developing comprehensive regulatory frameworks and safety standards is essential to manage the risks associated with nanotechnology while fostering innovation. Balancing these aspects is key to ensuring that the benefits of nanotechnology are realized without compromising environmental integrity or public safety. The environmental implications of nanotechnology are a growing area of research, as the introduction of nanomaterials into ecosystems raises concerns about their long-term effects. Nanomaterials can enter the environment through various pathways, including agricultural runoff, industrial waste, and the degradation of nanomaterial-containing products [54]. Once in the environment, these materials may interact with natural processes in complex ways. For example, nanoparticles may bind to soil particles, influence microbial communities, or be taken up by plants, potentially entering the food chain [55]. Understanding these interactions is crucial, as nanomaterials could have both positive and negative effects on ecosystems. On one hand, they could improve soil fertility and plant growth by enhancing nutrient availability. On the other hand, they could pose risks by disrupting soil and aquatic ecosystems, harming beneficial organisms, or accumulating in higher trophic levels. For instance, while some nanomaterials might help in pollutant remediation or improve soil health, others could be toxic to aquatic life, inhibit plant growth, or disrupt microbial activity [56]. Research has shown that certain nanoparticles, such as silver or titanium dioxide, can accumulate in the environment and cause harm to organisms, ranging from algae to fish. These potential risks underscore the importance of thorough environmental assessments that evaluate the lifecycle of nanomaterials—from production and use to disposal—and their cumulative impact on ecosystems. Given the potential risks associated with nanotechnology, robust regulatory frameworks and safety standards are essential to ensure that its development and application are safe for both the environment and public health. Regulatory bodies worldwide, including the U.S. Environmental Protection Agency (EPA), the European Chemicals Agency (ECHA), and various national agencies, are working to develop guidelines and regulations specific to nanomaterials [57]. These frameworks typically require manufacturers to provide detailed information on the chemical composition, environmental fate, and toxicity of nanomaterials before they are approved for commercial use. One of the challenges in regulating nanotechnology is the diversity and complexity of nanomaterials, which can vary widely in terms of size, shape, surface properties, and reactivity. This variability makes it difficult to establish one-size-fits-all safety standards. As a result, regulatory agencies are adopting a case-by-case approach, where each nanomaterial is assessed individually based on its specific properties and intended use. The dynamic nature of nanotechnology means that regulatory frameworks must be adaptable, incorporating the latest scientific findings and technological advancements [58]. Safety standards also extend to the labeling and handling of nanomaterials, ensuring that workers and consumers are informed about potential risks and safe usage practices. For example, in the European Union, the REACH (Registration, Evaluation, Authorisation, and Restriction of Chemicals) regulation requires detailed safety information for substances produced or imported in large quantities, including those at the nanoscale. This information helps to ensure that nanomaterials are used in a way that minimizes risk and protects both human health and the environment.

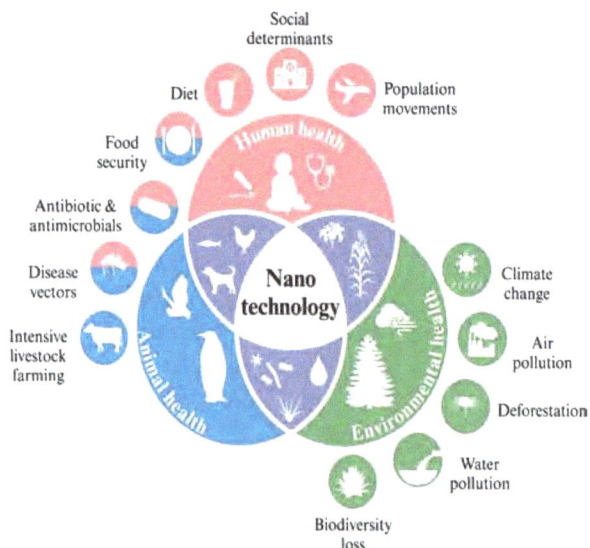

Fig. (1.2). Role of nanotechnology in maintaining the balance between human, animal & environmental health.

CONCLUSION AND FUTURE PERSPECTIVE

Nanotechnology in agriculture and food represents a transformative frontier that holds immense potential for addressing some of the most pressing challenges in modern agriculture and food security. Through the application of nanoscale materials and technologies, we can enhance crop yields, improve the precision of nutrient and pesticide delivery, extend the shelf life of food products, and ensure food safety through advanced monitoring systems. The innovations discussed, such as nanofertilizers, nanosensors, nanocoatings, and smart delivery systems, are not only improving the efficiency and sustainability of agricultural practices but are also leading to more nutritious, safer, and higher-quality food products. Moreover, the integration of nanotechnology in animal husbandry is helping to improve animal health and productivity, while also advancing veterinary medicine. However, as with any emerging technology, the widespread adoption of nanotechnology in agriculture and food must be approached with careful consideration of its environmental and societal impacts. The potential risks posed by nanomaterials to ecosystems, human health, and the broader environment necessitate thorough assessment and the development of robust regulatory frameworks. Ensuring that nanotechnology is deployed safely and ethically will be critical to its long-term success and acceptance by consumers and stakeholders. The continued advancement of nanotechnology in agriculture and food promises even greater innovations. As research progresses, we can expect to see more refined and efficient nanomaterials, new applications that further enhance sustainability, and improvements in the traceability and transparency of food supply chains. Additionally, interdisciplinary collaborations between scientists, engineers, policymakers, and industry leaders will be essential in driving forward the responsible development and implementation of these technologies.

REFERENCES

[1]   Jampílek, J.; Kráľová, K. Application Of nanotechnology in agriculture and food industry, its prospects and risks. *Ecol. Chem. Eng. S,* **2015**, *22*(3), 321-361.
       [http://dx.doi.org/10.1515/eces-2015-0018]

[2]   Sekhon, B. Nanotechnology in agri-food production: an overview. *Nanotechnol. Sci. Appl.,* **2014**, *7*, 31-53.
       [http://dx.doi.org/10.2147/NSA.S39406] [PMID: 24966671]

[3]   Tsouros, D.C.; Bibi, S.; Sarigiannidis, P.G. A Review on UAV-Based Applications for Precision Agriculture. *Information (Basel),* **2019**, *10*(11), 349.
       [http://dx.doi.org/10.3390/info10110349]

[4]   Movassaghian, S.; Merkel, O.M.; Torchilin, V.P. Applications of polymer micelles for imaging and drug delivery. *Wiley Interdiscip. Rev. Nanomed. Nanobiotechnol.,* **2015**, *7*(5), 691-707.
       [http://dx.doi.org/10.1002/wnan.1332] [PMID: 25683687]

[5]   Bhaskar, R.K.; Kumaraswamy, B. Nanotechnology based water purification systems for rural communities. *Nanotechnol. Percept.,* **2024**, *20*(S2)
       [http://dx.doi.org/10.62441/nano-ntp.v20iS2.87]

[6]   Duncan, T.V. Applications of nanotechnology in food packaging and food safety: Barrier materials, antimicrobials and sensors. *J. Colloid Interface Sci.,* **2011**, *363*(1), 1-24.
        [http://dx.doi.org/10.1016/j.jcis.2011.07.017] [PMID: 21824625]

[7]   Kah, M.; Kookana, R.S.; Gogos, A.; Bucheli, T.D. A critical evaluation of nanopesticides and nanofertilizers against their conventional analogues. *Nat. Nanotechnol.,* **2018**, *13*(8), 677-684.
        [http://dx.doi.org/10.1038/s41565-018-0131-1] [PMID: 29736032]

[8]   Ram, P.; Vivek, K.; Kumar, S.P. Nanotechnology in sustainable agriculture: Present concerns and future aspects. *Afr. J. Biotechnol.,* **2014**, *13*(6), 705-713.
        [http://dx.doi.org/10.5897/AJBX2013.13554]

[9]   Jasrotia, P.; Nagpal, M.; Mishra, C.N.; Sharma, A.K.; Kumar, S.; Kamble, U.; Bhardwaj, A.K.; Kashyap, P.L.; Kumar, S.; Singh, G.P. Nanomaterials for postharvest management of insect pests: Current state and future perspectives. *Frontiers in Nanotechnology,* **2022**, *3*, 811056.
        [http://dx.doi.org/10.3389/fnano.2021.811056]

[10]   Rhim, J.W.; Park, H.M.; Ha, C.S. Bio-nanocomposites for food packaging applications. *Prog. Polym. Sci.,* **2013**, *38*(10-11), 1629-1652.
        [http://dx.doi.org/10.1016/j.progpolymsci.2013.05.008]

[11]   Evrendilek, G.A.; R Richter, E. Concurrent detection of foodborne pathogens: past efforts and recent trends. *Journal of Food: Microbiology, Safety & Hygiene,* **2017**, *2*(1).
        [http://dx.doi.org/10.4172/2476-2059.1000116]

[12]   Yu, H.; Park, J.Y.; Kwon, C.W.; Hong, S.C.; Park, K.M.; Chang, P.S. An overview of nanotechnology in food science: preparative methods, practical applications, and safety. *J. Chem.,* **2018**, *2018*, 1-10.
        [http://dx.doi.org/10.1155/2018/5427978]

[13]   Sefton, M.V. Controlled release delivery systems. *J. Control. Release,* **1986**, *4*(1), 69-70.
        [http://dx.doi.org/10.1016/0168-3659(86)90036-2]

[14]   Ortman, K.; Pehrson, B. Selenite and selenium yeast as feed supplements for dairy cows. *J. Vet. Med. A,* **1997**, *44*(1–10), 373-380.
        [http://dx.doi.org/10.1111/j.1439-0442.1997.tb01121.x]

[15]   Porter, M.E.; Linde, C. Toward a New Conception of the Environment-Competitiveness Relationship. *J. Econ. Perspect.,* **1995**, *9*(4), 97-118.
        [http://dx.doi.org/10.1257/jep.9.4.97]

[16]   Ashitha A, Rakhimol KR. Fate of the conventional fertilizers in environment. *In Controlled-release fertilizers for sustainable agriculture,* **2021**; *1* pp. 25-39.
        [http://dx.doi.org/10.1016/B978-0-12-819555-0.00002-9]

[17]   Dhoundiyal, S.; Kaur, A.; Alam, M. A.; Sharma, A. the Future of Nanopesticides, Nanoherbicides, and Nanofertilizers. *CRC Press,* **2023**.
        [http://dx.doi.org/10.1201/9781003364429]

[18]   Monreal, C.M.; DeRosa, M.; Mallubhotla, S.C.; Bindraban, P.S.; Dimkpa, C. Nanotechnologies for increasing the crop use efficiency of fertilizer-micronutrients. *Biol. Fertil. Soils,* **2016**, *52*(3), 423-437.
        [http://dx.doi.org/10.1007/s00374-015-1073-5]

[19]   Kim, H.J.; Kim, T.; Lee, M. Responsive nanostructures from aqueous assembly of rigid-flexible block molecules. *Acc. Chem. Res.,* **2011**, *44*(1), 72-82.
        [http://dx.doi.org/10.1021/ar100111n] [PMID: 21128602]

[20]   Montalvo, D.; McLaughlin, M.J.; Degryse, F. Efficacy of Hydroxyapatite Nanoparticles as Phosphorus Fertilizer in Andisols and Oxisols. *Soil Sci. Soc. Am. J.,* **2015**, *79*(2), 551-558.
        [http://dx.doi.org/10.2136/sssaj2014.09.0373]

[21]   Joy, M.M.; Rammig, F.J. A hybrid methodology to detect memory leaks in soft real-time embedded systems software. *International Journal of Embedded Systems,* **2017**, *9*(1), 61.

[http://dx.doi.org/10.1504/IJES.2017.081723]

[22] Hood, E. Nanotechnology: looking as we leap. *Environ. Health Perspect.,* **2004**, *112*(13), A740-A749.
[http://dx.doi.org/10.1289/ehp.112-a740] [PMID: 15345364]

[23] Altieri, M.A. The ecological role of biodiversity in agroecosystems. *Agric. Ecosyst. Environ.,* **1999**, *74*(1-3), 19-31.
[http://dx.doi.org/10.1016/S0167-8809(99)00028-6]

[24] Singh, R.K.; Berkvens, R.; Weyn, M. AgriFusion: An Architecture for IoT and Emerging Technologies Based on a Precision Agriculture Survey. *IEEE Access,* **2021**, *9*, 136253-136283.
[http://dx.doi.org/10.1109/ACCESS.2021.3116814]

[25] Klaine, S.J.; Koelmans, A.A.; Horne, N.; Carley, S.; Handy, R.D.; Kapustka, L.; Nowack, B.; von der Kammer, F. Paradigms to assess the environmental impact of manufactured nanomaterials. *Environ. Toxicol. Chem.,* **2012**, *31*(1), 3-14.
[http://dx.doi.org/10.1002/etc.733] [PMID: 22162122]

[26] Lin, D.; Xing, B. Phytotoxicity of nanoparticles: Inhibition of seed germination and root growth. *Environ. Pollut.,* **2007**, *150*(2), 243-250.
[http://dx.doi.org/10.1016/j.envpol.2007.01.016] [PMID: 17374428]

[27] Environmental Fate and Risks of Nano-enabled Pesticides. *Chem. Int.,* **2017**, *39*(1).
[http://dx.doi.org/10.1515/ci-2017-0113]

[28] Monteiro, A.; Santos, S. Sustainable Approach to Weed Management: The Role of Precision Weed Management. *Agronomy (Basel),* **2022**, *12*(1), 118.
[http://dx.doi.org/10.3390/agronomy12010118]

[29] Manning, P.; Taylor, G.; Hanley, E.; Bioenergy, M. Food Production and Biodiversity - an Unlikely Alliance? *Glob. Change Biol. Bioenergy,* **2014**, *7*(4), 570-576.
[http://dx.doi.org/10.1111/gcbb.12173]

[30] Rhim, J.W.; Park, H.M.; Ha, C.S. Bio-nanocomposites for food packaging applications. *Prog. Polym. Sci.,* **2013**, *38*(10-11), 1629-1652.
[http://dx.doi.org/10.1016/j.progpolymsci.2013.05.008]

[31] Laufer, G.; Kirkland, C.; Cain, A.A.; Grunlan, J.C. Clay-chitosan nanobrick walls: completely renewable gas barrier and flame-retardant nanocoatings. *ACS Appl. Mater. Interfaces,* **2012**, *4*(3), 1643-1649.
[http://dx.doi.org/10.1021/am2017915] [PMID: 22339671]

[32] Theobald, D.L. How Industry Can Help Maintain a Healthy Environment. *J. Am. Water Works Assoc.,* **2014**, *106*(2), 69-71.
[http://dx.doi.org/10.5942/jawwa.2014.106.0031]

[33] Onwude, D.I.; Chen, G.; Eke-emezie, N.; Kabutey, A.; Khaled, A.Y.; Sturm, B. Recent Advances in Reducing Food Losses in the Supply Chain of Fresh Agricultural Produce. *Processes (Basel),* **2020**, *8*(11), 1431.
[http://dx.doi.org/10.3390/pr8111431]

[34] Silvestre, C.; Duraccio, D.; Cimmino, S. Food packaging based on polymer nanomaterials. *Prog. Polym. Sci.,* **2011**, *36*(12), 1766-1782.
[http://dx.doi.org/10.1016/j.progpolymsci.2011.02.003]

[35] Ferrari, M. Cancer nanotechnology: opportunities and challenges. *Nat. Rev. Cancer,* **2005**, *5*(3), 161-171.
[http://dx.doi.org/10.1038/nrc1566] [PMID: 15738981]

[36] Luk'yanchuk, B.; Zheludev, N.I.; Maier, S.A.; Halas, N.J.; Nordlander, P.; Giessen, H.; Chong, C.T. The Fano resonance in plasmonic nanostructures and metamaterials. *Nat. Mater.,* **2010**, *9*(9), 707-715.
[http://dx.doi.org/10.1038/nmat2810] [PMID: 20733610]

[37] Medintz, I.L.; Clapp, A.R.; Mattoussi, H.; Goldman, E.R.; Fisher, B.; Mauro, J.M. Self-assembled nanoscale biosensors based on quantum dot FRET donors. *Nat. Mater.,* **2003**, *2*(9), 630-638.
[http://dx.doi.org/10.1038/nmat961] [PMID: 12942071]

[38] Fraceto, L.F.; Grillo, R.; de Medeiros, G.A.; Scognamiglio, V.; Rea, G.; Bartolucci, C. Nanotechnology in Agriculture: Which Innovation Potential Does It Have? *Front. Environ. Sci.,* **2016**, *4*.
[http://dx.doi.org/10.3389/fenvs.2016.00020]

[39] Leung, W.H.; Zou, L.; Lo, W.H.; Chan, P.H. An Amyloid-Fibril-Based Colorimetric Nanosensor for Rapid and Sensitive Chromium(VI) Detection. *ChemPlusChem,* **2013**, *78*(12), 1440-1445.
[http://dx.doi.org/10.1002/cplu.201300267] [PMID: 31986653]

[40] Huang, X.J.; Choi, Y.K. Chemical sensors based on nanostructured materials. *Sens. Actuators B Chem.,* **2007**, *122*(2), 659-671.
[http://dx.doi.org/10.1016/j.snb.2006.06.022]

[41] Qin, J.; Chen, H. Using Genetic Algorithm in Building Domain-Specific Collections: An Experiment in the Nanotechnology Domain, **2005**.
[http://dx.doi.org/10.1109/HICSS.2005.659]

[42] Armenta, R.E.; Valentine, M.C. Single-Cell Oils as a Source of Omega-3 Fatty Acids: An Overview of Recent Advances. *J. Am. Oil Chem. Soc.,* **2013**, *90*(2), 167-182.
[http://dx.doi.org/10.1007/s11746-012-2154-3]

[43] Mu, P. *Sequence-Defined Molecules Can Be Used to Create 2D Nanomaterials*; Science Trends, **2018**.
[http://dx.doi.org/10.31988/SciTrends.42065]

[44] Weiss, J.; Takhistov, P.; McClements, D.J. Functional Materials in Food Nanotechnology. *J. Food Sci.,* **2006**, *71*(9), R107-R116.
[http://dx.doi.org/10.1111/j.1750-3841.2006.00195.x]

[45] Godfray, H.C.J.; Beddington, J.R.; Crute, I.R.; Haddad, L.; Lawrence, D.; Muir, J.F.; Pretty, J.; Robinson, S.; Thomas, S.M.; Toulmin, C. Food security: the challenge of feeding 9 billion people. *Science,* **2010**, *327*(5967), 812-818.
[http://dx.doi.org/10.1126/science.1185383] [PMID: 20110467]

[46] Manzocco, L.; Mikkonen, K.S.; García-González, C.A. Aerogels as porous structures for food applications: Smart ingredients and novel packaging materials. *Food Struct.,* **2021**, *28*, 100188.
[http://dx.doi.org/10.1016/j.foostr.2021.100188]

[47] Gomes, C.; Moreira, R.G.; Castell-Perez, E. Poly (DL-lactide-co-glycolide) (PLGA) nanoparticles with entrapped trans-cinnamaldehyde and eugenol for antimicrobial delivery applications. *J. Food Sci.,* **2011**, *76*(2), N16-N24.
[http://dx.doi.org/10.1111/j.1750-3841.2010.01985.x] [PMID: 21535781]

[48] Tian, L. Development of a sensor-based precision herbicide application system. *Comput. Electron. Agric.,* **2002**, *36*(2-3), 133-149.
[http://dx.doi.org/10.1016/S0168-1699(02)00097-2]

[49] Pidgeon, N.; Rogers-Hayden, T. Opening up nanotechnology dialogue with the publics: Risk communication or 'upstream engagement'? *Health Risk Soc.,* **2007**, *9*(2), 191-210.
[http://dx.doi.org/10.1080/13698570701306906]

[50] Sounkaria, S.; Chandra, P. Ovarian Cancer: Potential biomarkers and nanotechnology based diagnostic tools. *Adv. Nat. Sci.: Nanosci. Nanotechnol.,* **2021**, *12*(3), 033001.
[http://dx.doi.org/10.1088/2043-6262/ac2741]

[51] Husni, P.; Ramadhania, Z.M. Plant Extract Loaded Nanoparticles. *Indones. J. Pharm.,* **2021**, *3*(1), 38.
[http://dx.doi.org/10.24198/idjp.v3i1.34032]

[52] Saleh, T. A. Trends in nanomaterial types, synthesis methods, properties and uses: toxicity,

environmental concerns and economic viability. *Nano-structures & Nano-objects,* **2024**, *37*, 101109-101109.
[http://dx.doi.org/10.1016/j.nanoso.2024.101109]

[53] Yang, C.C.; Mai, Y.W. Thermodynamics at the nanoscale: A new approach to the investigation of unique physicochemical properties of nanomaterials. *Mater. Sci. Eng. Rep.,* **2014**, *79*, 1-40.
[http://dx.doi.org/10.1016/j.mser.2014.02.001]

[54] Lin, Y.X.; Gao, Y.J.; Wang, Y.; Qiao, Z.Y.; Fan, G.; Qiao, S.L.; Zhang, R.X.; Wang, L.; Wang, H. pH-sensitive polymeric nanoparticles with gold(I) compound payloads synergistically induce cancer cell death through modulation of autophagy. *Mol. Pharm.,* **2015**, *12*(8), 2869-2878.
[http://dx.doi.org/10.1021/acs.molpharmaceut.5b00060] [PMID: 26101892]

[55] Shah, V.; Belozerova, I. Influence of metal nanoparticles on the soil microbial community and germination of lettuce seeds. *Water Air Soil Pollut.,* **2009**, *197*(1-4), 143-148.
[http://dx.doi.org/10.1007/s11270-008-9797-6]

[56] Barrena, R.; Casals, E.; Colón, J.; Font, X.; Sánchez, A.; Puntes, V. Evaluation of the ecotoxicity of model nanoparticles. *Chemosphere,* **2009**, *75*(7), 850-857.
[http://dx.doi.org/10.1016/j.chemosphere.2009.01.078] [PMID: 19264345]

[57] Jennings, A.A. Worldwide regulatory guidance values for surface soil exposure to noncarcinogenic polycyclic aromatic hydrocarbons. *J. Environ. Manage.,* **2012**, *101*, 173-190.
[http://dx.doi.org/10.1016/j.jenvman.2012.02.011] [PMID: 22446072]

[58] Kah, M.; Tufenkji, N.; White, J.C. Nano-enabled strategies to enhance crop nutrition and protection. *Nat. Nanotechnol.,* **2019**, *14*(6), 532-540.
[http://dx.doi.org/10.1038/s41565-019-0439-5] [PMID: 31168071]

CHAPTER 2

Nanotechnology in Everyday Cosmetics

Abstract: This chapter provides a comprehensive exploration of the role of nanotechnology in cosmetics, beginning with an overview of nano-cosmetics and their evolution within the industry. The use of nanomaterials, such as nanoparticles, nanoemulsions, liposomes, and niosomes, has enabled the development of advanced delivery systems that significantly improve the penetration, absorption, and targeted delivery of active ingredients. These innovations have resulted in products with improved stability, extended shelf life, and enhanced skin hydration and protection, elevating the performance and appeal of cosmetic products. The chapter talks about the critical safety and regulatory aspects of nano-cosmetics. As the incorporation of nanomaterials raises toxicological concerns, thorough safety assessments are essential to ensure consumer protection. Regulatory frameworks and guidelines, including those from the FDA, EMA, and international standards, are discussed to highlight the measures taken to ensure the safe use of nano-cosmetics. Additionally, consumer safety and awareness are emphasized as crucial components in the responsible development and marketing of these products. The chapter examines how the rapid growth of the nano-cosmetics market is driven by consumer demand for innovative and effective beauty solutions. Consumer perceptions and preferences are evolving as awareness of nanotechnology increases, influencing purchasing decisions and brand loyalty, and addressing the ethical considerations and sustainability challenges associated with the production and disposal of nano-cosmetics, emphasizing the need for responsible practices in the industry.

Keywords: Awareness, Cosmetics, Market, Personal care, Regulatory frameworks, Safety.

INTRODUCTION

Nano-cosmetics are at the cutting edge of the beauty and personal care industry, revolutionizing traditional formulations by incorporating nanotechnology to enhance product efficacy, texture, and user experience. The essence of nanotechnology lies in its ability to manipulate materials at the nanoscale—dimensions so small that they operate on the same scale as biological molecules [1]. This size manipulation imparts unique properties to ingredients, such as increased surface area, enhanced solubility, and improved skin penetration. In cosmetics, these properties are harnessed to create products that deliver active ingredients more effectively to the targeted areas, leading to improved skin hydration, anti-aging effects, and protection against environmental stressors. For instance, nano-sized particles in sunscreens not only offer superior UV protection but also ensure a more even application, avoiding the pasty appearance associated with traditional sunscreens [2]. Additionally, nano-cosmetics include anti-aging serums, where nano-encapsulated vitamins and antioxidants penetrate deeper skin layers, promoting cellular repair and rejuvenation. The scope of nano-cosmetics also extends to hair care, where nanoparticles help in delivering nutrients directly to hair follicles, enhancing hair strength and shine. The advent of nano-cosmetics signifies a paradigm shift towards more personalized and effective skincare solutions, driven by scientific innovation at the molecular level. The evolution of nanotechnology in the cosmetic industry is a testament to the relentless quest for innovation and improved product performance. The journey began with basic applications, such as the introduction of nano-sized titanium dioxide and zinc oxide in sunscreens, which provided not only superior UV protection but also a more aesthetically pleasing application, free of the white cast that was a common complaint with traditional formulations [3]. These early successes sparked interest and investment in the broader application of nanotechnology across various cosmetic products. As research progressed, the industry witnessed the development of more sophisticated nanocarriers such as liposomes, niosomes, and solid lipid nanoparticles. These carriers were designed to encapsulate active ingredients, protecting them from environmental degradation and enhancing their delivery to deeper skin layers, thus maximizing their therapeutic effects. The ability to control the release of active ingredients over time became a key innovation, allowing for sustained efficacy and reduced application frequency. Moreover, the cosmetic industry has embraced nanoemulsions, which offer improved texture and stability in products, enhancing consumer satisfaction. The evolution of nanotechnology in cosmetics is also marked by a growing emphasis on safety and regulation, as the industry recognizes the need to balance innovation with consumer safety.

FORMULATION AND EFFICACY OF NANO-COSMETICS

Nano-cosmetics use nanotechnology to create advanced skin care products with enhanced effectiveness, stability, and user experience, as listed in Table **2.1**. By reducing ingredients to nanoscale sizes, these products allow deeper skin penetration and better delivery of active ingredients like vitamins and antioxidants. Nano-encapsulation protects sensitive ingredients from degradation, leading to a longer shelf-life and consistent performance [4]. The small size of nanoparticles also improves the texture and feel of the products, offering smoother, non-greasy formulations. Overall, nano-cosmetics provide superior results, addressing various skin concerns with greater efficiency and consumer satisfaction.

Table 2.1. Different types of nanomaterials commonly used in cosmetic products.

Type of Nanomaterial	Description	Application	Benefits	Examples	References
Nanoparticles	Solid particles sized between 1-100 nm, often made of metals, metal oxides, or polymers.	Used in sunscreens, anti-aging creams, and color cosmetics.	Enhanced UV protection, better coverage, and improved skin adhesion.	Zinc oxide and titanium dioxide nanoparticles in sunscreens.	[5]
Nanoemulsions	Fine oil-in-water or water-in-oil emulsions with droplet sizes in the nanometer range.	Found in moisturizers, lotions, and hair care products.	Improved delivery of active ingredients, increased skin penetration, and enhanced texture.	Nanoemulsion-based moisturizers for deep skin hydration.	[6]
Liposomes	Spherical vesicles with a phospholipid bilayer, capable of encapsulating active ingredients.	Commonly used in anti-aging creams, serums, and drug delivery systems.	Targeted delivery, controlled release, reduced irritation potential, and increased ingredient stability.	Liposome-based anti-aging serums.	[7]
Niosomes	Non-ionic surfactant vesicles, similar to liposomes but more stable and cost-effective.	Used in skincare products for moisturization and targeted delivery.	Enhanced penetration, stability, and controlled release of active ingredients.	Niosome-encapsulated vitamin C serums.	[8]
Dendrimers	Highly branched, tree-like polymeric nanostructures with a high degree of functionality.	Utilized in anti-aging products and delivery systems for active ingredients.	Precision in drug delivery, high loading capacity, and sustained release.	Dendrimer-based anti-aging treatments.	[9]

(Table 2.1) cont.....

Type of Nanomaterial	Description	Application	Benefits	Examples	References
Nanocrystals	Crystalline particles with sizes in the nanometer range, often used to enhance solubility.	Applied in anti-aging products, sunscreens, and whitening agents.	Increased bioavailability, enhanced UV protection, improved skin lightening effects.	Nanocrystal-based skin whitening creams.	[10]
Fullerenes	Carbon-based nanomaterials shaped like hollow spheres, tubes, or ellipsoids.	Incorporated in anti-aging and antioxidant formulations.	Strong antioxidant properties, protection against free radicals, and anti-aging effects.	Fullerene-enriched anti-aging creams.	[11]
Nanogels	Hydrated polymer networks on a nanoscale, used for delivering active ingredients.	Found in moisturizers, anti-aging products, and wound care.	Improved hydration, controlled release, and targeted delivery of active compounds.	Nanogel-based wound healing creams.	[12]
Nanocapsules	Capsules with a core-shell structure encapsulating active ingredients for targeted delivery.	Used in anti-aging products and sensitive skin formulations.	Protection of active ingredients, controlled release, and enhanced stability.	Nanocapsule-based retinol serums	[13]
Nanofibers	Ultra-fine fibers with a diameter in the nanometer range, used in advanced delivery systems.	Applied in wound care, facial masks, and transdermal patches.	Increased surface area, controlled release, and enhanced absorption.	Nanofiber-based facial masks.	[14]

Types of Nanomaterials Used in Cosmetics

Nanomaterials have become integral to the cosmetic industry, offering unique properties that traditional ingredients can't match. These materials, engineered at the nanoscale, exhibit enhanced physical, chemical, and biological characteristics that improve the efficacy and sensory experience of cosmetic products. Titanium dioxide (TiO_2) and zinc oxide (ZnO) nanoparticles are commonly used in sunscreens for their ability to provide broad-spectrum UV protection without leaving a white residue, making them ideal for sensitive skin. Silver nanoparticles are valued for their antimicrobial properties, often used in acne treatments to reduce bacteria on the skin [15]. Gold nanoparticles, known for their anti-aging benefits, are used to stimulate collagen production, reduce wrinkles, and enhance the delivery of other active ingredients in luxury skincare products. Nanoemulsions, particularly lipid-based and polymeric varieties, are used to improve the delivery and penetration of active ingredients, such as vitamins and antioxidants, into the skin. These nanoemulsions are often found in moisturizers and anti-aging creams, where they ensure a more effective and sustained release of beneficial compounds. Nanocapsules, another form of nanotechnology, are designed to encapsulate and protect sensitive active ingredients from degradation, ensuring their stability and enhancing their efficacy [16]. This technology allows for targeted delivery, directing ingredients to specific areas of the skin for optimal results. Fullerenes, a class of carbon-based nanomaterials, are renowned for their potent antioxidant properties, making them valuable in anti-aging and skin protection products. These materials help neutralize free radicals and protect the skin from environmental stressors like pollution and UV radiation. Nanoclays, such as bentonite and kaolin, are used in face masks and mattifying products for their oil-absorbing capabilities, particularly beneficial for those with oily or acne-prone skin [17]. While these advancements in nanotechnology have led to more effective and long-lasting cosmetic products, they also raise concerns about safety and regulation, as the long-term impacts on human health and the environment are still being studied. Nanotechnology's role in cosmetics continues to evolve, with ongoing research and development pushing the boundaries of what these tiny materials can achieve. Liposomes, for example, are spherical vesicles that can encapsulate active ingredients, such as peptides and vitamins, and deliver them deeper into the skin. This targeted delivery system not only increases the efficacy of the ingredients but also minimizes potential irritation, making liposomes a popular choice in sensitive skin formulations. Solid lipid nanoparticles (SLNs) and nanostructured lipid carriers (NLCs) are other advanced forms of lipid-based nanomaterials used in cosmetics [18]. These systems are designed to improve the stability and bioavailability of active ingredients, providing controlled release and enhanced skin hydration. They are particularly useful in anti-aging creams, sunscreens, and moisturizers. As the cosmetic industry continues to embrace nanotechnology, there is a growing emphasis on research and development to create safer, more effective, and environmentally friendly products. The dynamic nature of nanotechnology allows for continuous innovation, leading to new applications that go beyond traditional cosmetic functions. For example, nanoemulsions are being increasingly used for their ability to deliver hydrophobic active ingredients, such as vitamins and essential oils, in a stable, water-based formulation [19]. This not only enhances the sensory properties of cosmetic products but also improves the penetration and absorption of active ingredients, offering consumers more immediate and noticeable results. Nanoparticles like titanium dioxide and zinc oxide are widely used in sunscreens due to their ability to provide broad-spectrum UV protection without leaving a white residue on the skin, as depicted in Fig. (**2.1**). These nanoparticles are transparent to visible light, making them ideal for daily use in cosmetic formulations, as they blend seamlessly into the skin while providing robust protection against harmful UV rays [20]. Moreover, these nanomaterials are engineered to stay on the skin's surface, minimizing the risk of deep penetration and potential adverse effects. Another promising development in nano-cosmetics is the use of nanocarriers for the controlled release of fragrances. By encapsulating fragrance molecules in nanoparticles, cosmetic companies can create products that release scent over time, providing a long-lasting fragrance experience without the need for reapplication. This technology also protects sensitive fragrance compounds from degradation, ensuring that the scent remains fresh and potent for longer periods. Despite the clear benefits, the use of nanotechnology in cosmetics has prompted ongoing discussions about its long-term safety and environmental sustainability. Researchers and industry stakeholders are collaborating to develop comprehensive testing protocols and guidelines that address these concerns. The focus is on understanding the interaction of nanomaterials with biological systems and the environment, ensuring that their use in cosmetics is both safe for consumers and sustainable for the planet. As consumers become more aware of the potential benefits and risks associated with nanotechnology, transparency in product labeling and communication becomes essential. Brands that prioritize transparency and provide detailed information about the nanomaterials used in their products are likely to build greater trust and loyalty among consumers.

Enhanced Delivery Systems

The integration of nanotechnology into cosmetic formulations has revolutionized the delivery systems used in skincare and beauty products. Enhanced delivery systems in nano-cosmetics are designed to improve the effectiveness of active ingredients by optimizing their stability, penetration, and bioavailability. These systems utilize nanomaterials such as liposomes, solid lipid nanoparticles, and nanoemulsions, which are engineered to encapsulate active compounds and protect them from degradation while ensuring their controlled release over time. One of the most significant advantages of nanotechnology in cosmetics is its ability to enhance the penetration and absorption of active ingredients into the skin. Traditional cosmetic formulations often struggle with delivering ingredients past the skin's outermost layer, the stratum corneum [21]. Nanoparticles, due to their small size, can penetrate deeper into the skin layers, reaching the epidermis and dermis, where they can exert their intended effects more efficiently. For example, in anti-aging products, nanoparticles can carry antioxidants, vitamins, or peptides directly to the deeper skin layers, where they can stimulate collagen production, reduce oxidative stress, and improve skin elasticity, as depicted in Fig. (**2.2**) [22]. This targeted delivery not only enhances the efficacy of the ingredients but also minimizes potential side effects by ensuring that the active compounds are delivered precisely where they are needed, rather than being spread across the skin's surface. The encapsulation of hydrophobic (water-insoluble) ingredients within nanoparticles allows these substances to be delivered in a stable, water-based formulation. This improves their solubility and bioavailability, making them more effective in lower concentrations [23]. The result is a more potent product that can deliver visible results with minimal irritation or adverse reactions, which is particularly beneficial for sensitive skin types. Nanotechnology also enables the targeted delivery of active ingredients, which is a game-changer in cosmetic science. This approach involves designing nanoparticles that can deliver their payloads to specific cells or tissues, reducing the likelihood of off-target effects and enhancing the overall effectiveness of the treatment. For instance, in anti-acne formulations, nanoparticles can be engineered to target sebaceous glands, delivering antibacterial or anti-inflammatory agents directly to the site of action. This targeted delivery ensures that the active ingredients are concentrated where they are most needed, reducing the risk of systemic side effects and improving treatment outcomes [24]. In addition, targeted delivery systems can be designed to respond to specific triggers in the skin, such as pH changes, temperature, or enzymatic activity. These stimuli-responsive nanoparticles can release their active ingredients only when they encounter specific conditions, providing a controlled release that maximizes the ingredient's efficacy and minimizes waste. This precision in delivery not only enhances the effectiveness of cosmetic treatments but also contributes to the sustainability of the product by reducing the amount of active ingredient required. The ability to deliver multiple active ingredients simultaneously through different types of nanoparticles opens up new possibilities for multifunctional products. For example, a single nano-cosmetic formulation can be designed to deliver hydrating agents, anti-aging compounds, and sun protection all in one, offering a comprehensive skincare solution that addresses multiple concerns with high efficiency [25].

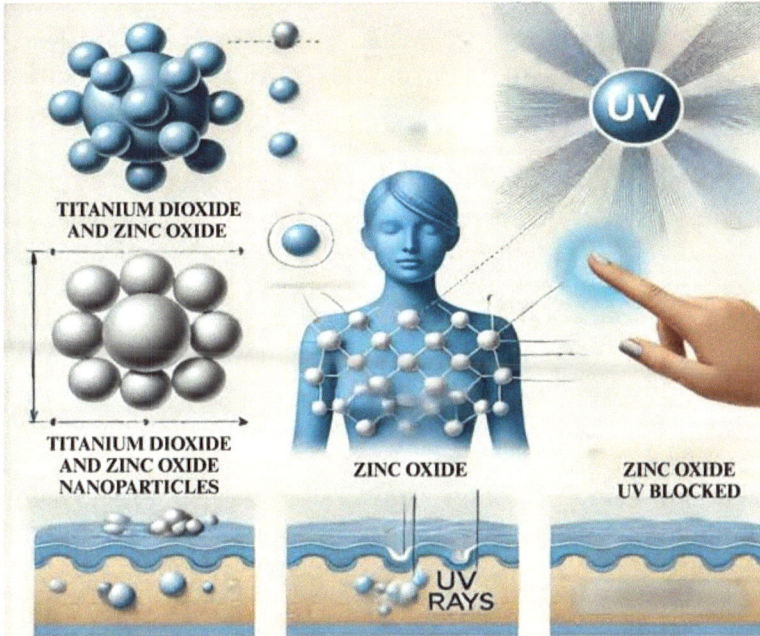

Fig. (2.1). Skin protection against UV rays by applying titanium dioxide or zinc oxide-based nanoparticles formulated in a sunscreen form.

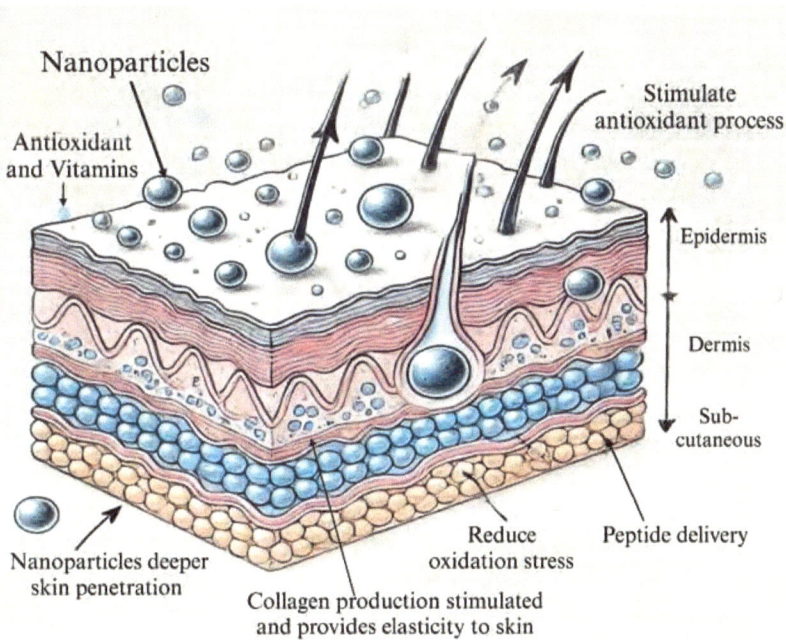

Fig. (2.2). Nanoparticles enhances skincare delivery.

Efficacy and Performance Benefits

The application of nanotechnology in the formulation of cosmetics brings substantial enhancements to the efficacy and performance of skincare and beauty products. By utilising the unique properties of nanoparticles, cosmetic formulations can deliver superior results in terms of stability, effectiveness, and user satisfaction, as depicted in Fig. (**2.3**). The efficacy of nano-cosmetics is reflected in their ability to improve the delivery and action of active ingredients, leading to noticeable benefits in skin appearance and health [26]. One of the key performance benefits of nano-cosmetics is the improved stability and extended shelf life of the products. Traditional cosmetic formulations often face challenges related to the stability of active ingredients, which can degrade over time due to exposure to light, air, and temperature fluctuations. This degradation not only reduces the effectiveness of the product but can also lead to changes in texture, color, and scent, ultimately affecting the overall user experience. Nanotechnology addresses these issues by encapsulating active ingredients within nanoparticles, which act as protective carriers. These nanoparticles are engineered to shield the active compounds from environmental factors that cause degradation [27]. For example, antioxidants such as vitamins C and E, which are prone to oxidation, can be encapsulated within lipid-based nanoparticles to protect them from exposure to air and light. This encapsulation not only preserves the potency of the active ingredients but also maintains the product's consistency and appearance over time. The controlled release properties of nanoparticles further contribute to product stability. By gradually releasing active ingredients over time, nano-cosmetics ensure a consistent delivery of benefits to the skin, even after prolonged storage. This controlled release mechanism also prevents the rapid degradation of sensitive ingredients, extending the shelf life of the product and ensuring that it remains effective for a longer period. The improved stability provided by nanotechnology allows for the reduction of preservatives and stabilizers in the formulation, which can be beneficial for consumers with sensitive skin or those seeking cleaner, more natural products. This enhancement in stability and shelf life is a significant advantage for both consumers and manufacturers, as it ensures that products remain effective and safe for use over an extended period, reducing waste and enhancing consumer trust [28].

Another critical aspect of the efficacy of nano-cosmetics is their ability to enhance skin hydration and protection. Nanoparticles can deliver moisturizing agents more effectively to the deeper layers of the skin, providing long-lasting hydration and improving overall skin health. Traditional moisturizers often struggle to penetrate beyond the skin's surface, leading to temporary hydration that fades quickly [29]. In contrast, nano-cosmetics can deliver hydrating ingredients such as hyaluronic acid, glycerine, and ceramides deep into the skin, where they can provide sustained moisture retention and reinforce the skin's natural barrier function. The ability of nanoparticles to enhance skin hydration is particularly beneficial for individuals with dry or sensitive skin, as it helps to restore the skin's moisture balance and alleviate discomfort associated with dryness. Additionally, by delivering active ingredients more efficiently, nano-cosmetics can reduce the need for frequent reapplication, providing long-lasting results and improving user satisfaction. In terms of skin protection, nano-cosmetics offer superior performance by incorporating UV filters and antioxidants into their formulations [30]. Nanoparticles can encapsulate and stabilize these protective agents, ensuring that they are evenly distributed across the skin and provide comprehensive coverage. For example, nano-sized zinc oxide and titanium dioxide particles are commonly used in sunscreens to provide broad-spectrum UV protection without leaving a white residue on the skin. The small size of these particles allows for better coverage and a more aesthetically pleasing finish, making sun protection more accessible and enjoyable for consumers. The inclusion of antioxidants in nano-cosmetics helps neutralize free radicals generated by UV exposure and environmental pollutants, preventing oxidative damage to the skin [31]. By delivering these protective agents deep into the skin, nano-cosmetics enhance the skin's resilience against external aggressors, reducing the risk of premature aging, hyperpigmentation, and other skin concerns.

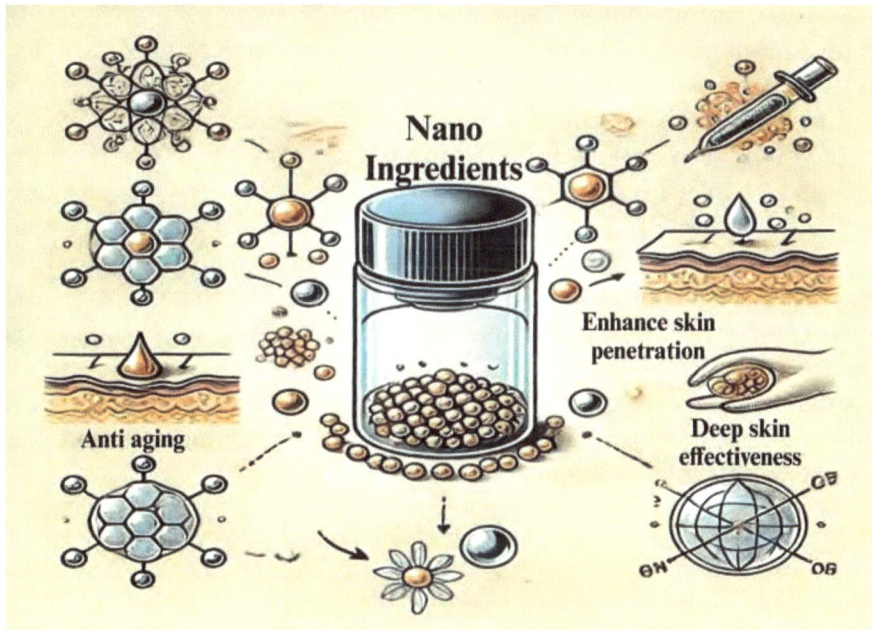

Fig. (2.3). Nanotechnology in improving the efficacy of cosmetics.

SAFETY AND REGULATORY ASPECTS

Nanotechnology in cosmetics has revolutionized the beauty industry, offering products with enhanced efficacy and innovative applications. However, the use of nanoparticles in cosmetic formulations also raises critical safety and regulatory concerns that must be meticulously addressed to ensure consumer protection and industry compliance [32]. This section dives into the toxicological considerations, regulatory frameworks, and consumer safety measures associated with nano-cosmetics.

The small size and unique properties of nanoparticles, which contribute to their effectiveness in cosmetic formulations, also pose potential risks that differ from those associated with conventional materials. Nanoparticles can penetrate the skin barrier more easily than larger particles, leading to concerns about their potential for systemic absorption, bioaccumulation, and toxicity [33]. Therefore, it is imperative to conduct thorough toxicological assessments to evaluate the safety of nano-cosmetics. Toxicological studies focus on understanding how nanoparticles interact with biological systems, including their potential to cause skin irritation, sensitization, or long-term health effects [34]. These studies often involve in vitro and in vivo testing to assess the cytotoxicity, genotoxicity, and immunotoxicity of nanoparticles. Researchers also examine the potential for nanoparticles to induce oxidative stress, inflammation, and DNA damage, which could contribute to adverse health outcomes. The physicochemical properties of nanoparticles, such as their size, shape, surface charge, and coating materials, play a crucial role in determining their safety profile. For example, smaller nanoparticles may have a higher potential for penetration and toxicity, while surface modifications can either mitigate or exacerbate their effects [35]. As such, safety assessments must consider these variables to accurately evaluate the risks associated with each specific type of nanoparticle used in cosmetics. In addition to direct toxicological concerns, there is also the need to consider the environmental impact of nano-cosmetics. The release of nanoparticles into the environment through wastewater can lead to their accumulation in ecosystems, where they may pose risks to aquatic organisms and other wildlife. Therefore, safety assessments must also address the potential environmental hazards of nano-cosmetics to ensure that their use does not compromise ecological health.

Given the complexities and potential risks associated with nano-cosmetics, regulatory authorities have established specific frameworks and guidelines to govern their development, production, and marketing. These regulations are designed to ensure that nano-cosmetics are safe for consumer use and that they comply with international standards for quality and safety. In the United States, the Food and Drug Administration (FDA) oversees the regulation of cosmetics, including those that incorporate nanotechnology [36]. The FDA requires manufacturers to ensure the safety of their products, including conducting appropriate safety testing for nanoparticles. While the FDA does not have specific regulations that differentiate nano-cosmetics from other cosmetics, it emphasizes the need for transparency and accurate labeling, particularly when nanoparticles are used. The European Medicines Agency (EMA), along with the European Union's Cosmetics Regulation (EC) No 1223/2009, provides a more comprehensive regulatory framework for nano-cosmetics. This regulation mandates that any cosmetic product containing nanoparticles must be clearly labeled and undergo a safety assessment by the Scientific Committee on Consumer Safety (SCCS) [37]. The SCCS evaluates the safety of nanoparticles used in cosmetics, considering their potential for dermal penetration and systemic exposure. Products that contain nanoparticles must be approved by the EMA before they can be marketed in the EU. Beyond the FDA and EMA, some international standards and guidelines govern the safety and regulation of nano-cosmetics. Organizations such as the International Organization for Standardization (ISO) and the Organization for Economic Co-operation and Development (OECD) have developed standards for the testing and assessment of nanomaterials [38]. These standards aim to harmonize safety testing methods and provide a consistent approach to evaluating the risks associated with nanoparticles in cosmetics. Compliance with these international standards is crucial for manufacturers who wish to market their products globally. It ensures that nano-cosmetics meet the safety and quality requirements of different regulatory jurisdictions and that consumers are protected from potential health risks. Adherence to these standards also fosters consumer confidence and trust in nano-cosmetics, as it demonstrates a commitment to safety and transparency.

Consumer safety is a paramount concern in the development and marketing of nano-cosmetics. Manufacturers must not only ensure that their products are safe but also educate consumers about the benefits and potential risks associated with nano-cosmetics. This involves clear and accurate labeling, which includes information about the presence of nanoparticles and any precautions that should be taken during use. Transparency is essential in building consumer trust. Providing detailed information about the types of nanoparticles used, their benefits, and the safety measures taken during product formulation can help alleviate consumer concerns [39]. Additionally, manufacturers should offer guidance on the proper use of nano-cosmetics, including instructions on application, storage, and disposal to minimize any potential risks. Public awareness campaigns and educational initiatives can also play a vital role in enhancing consumer safety. By informing consumers about the science behind nano-cosmetics, including the rigorous safety assessments and regulatory oversight they undergo, manufacturers can help dispel myths and misconceptions about nanotechnology. These efforts can empower consumers to make informed decisions about the products they use and to recognize the value of nano-cosmetics in enhancing their beauty and skincare routines.

MARKET TRENDS AND CONSUMER IMPACT

Nanotechnology has also significantly influenced market dynamics and consumer behavior. This section explores the rapid growth of the nano-cosmetics market, consumer perceptions and preferences, the ethical and sustainability considerations shaping the industry, and the future trends likely to dominate the landscape [40]. The nano-cosmetics market has witnessed substantial growth over the past decade, driven by advancements in nanotechnology and increasing consumer demand for high-performance beauty and skincare products, and such nano cosmetics products are listed in Table **2.2**. The unique capabilities of nanoparticles, such as enhanced skin penetration, targeted delivery, and prolonged release of active ingredients, have positioned nano-cosmetics as a premium segment within the broader cosmetics industry. This growth is further bolstered by the rising awareness among consumers about the benefits of nanotechnology in delivering superior cosmetic outcomes, such as improved hydration, anti-aging effects, and UV protection [41]. Market research indicates that the nano-cosmetics sector is expanding at a robust pace, with projections suggesting continued growth in the coming years. Factors contributing to this growth include increased investment in research and development, the introduction of innovative nano-based formulations, and the expansion of product lines to include a wider range of skincare, haircare, and color cosmetics. The growing trend of personalized skincare, where products are tailored to individual skin types and concerns, has been facilitated by the precision and versatility of nanotechnology [42]. The proliferation of e-commerce platforms has played a crucial role in the market's expansion, enabling consumers to access a diverse array of nano-cosmetic products from global brands. The ease of online shopping, combined with targeted digital marketing strategies, has made nano-cosmetics more accessible to a broader audience, further driving market growth. Consumer perceptions and preferences are pivotal in shaping the demand for nano-cosmetics. As consumers become more informed and discerning about the ingredients and technologies used in their beauty products, the appeal of nano-cosmetics has grown. Many consumers are attracted to the promise of enhanced efficacy, with nano-cosmetics often marketed as offering superior performance compared to traditional formulations. This includes claims of faster and more visible results, which resonate with consumers seeking effective solutions for skincare concerns such as aging, pigmentation, and acne [43]. Consumer perceptions are not uniformly positive. Some consumers express concerns about the safety and long-term effects of nanoparticles, fuelled by the broader debate on the safety of nanomaterials.

This has led to a segment of the market that is cautious or sceptical about using nano-cosmetics, particularly in regions where regulatory guidelines and safety assessments are less transparent or rigorous. To address these concerns, companies must emphasize transparency, providing clear information about the safety testing and regulatory compliance of their nano-cosmetic products. Preferences within the nano-cosmetics market are also influenced by cultural and regional factors. For example, in Asian markets, where skincare routines are deeply ingrained and often involve multiple steps, there is a strong preference for products that offer multifunctional benefits, such as moisturizing, brightening, and sun protection. Nano-cosmetics that deliver these combined effects are particularly popular in these regions [44]. In contrast, Western markets may prioritize anti-aging and anti-pollution properties, driving demand for nano-cosmetics that focus on these benefits. As the nano-cosmetics market grows, ethical considerations and sustainability have become increasingly important to both consumers and industry stakeholders. The production and use of nanomaterials raise several ethical questions, particularly regarding the environmental impact and the long-term health implications of nanoparticles [45]. The potential for nanoparticles to accumulate in the environment, particularly in aquatic ecosystems, has led to concerns about their impact on biodiversity and ecological balance. As a result, there is a growing demand for eco-friendly and sustainable nano-cosmetics that minimize environmental harm. Sustainability in nano-cosmetics is also closely linked to the sourcing of raw materials and the production processes used [46]. Consumers are increasingly seeking products that are not only effective but also align with their values of environmental responsibility and social ethics. This has driven the demand for sustainably sourced ingredients, cruelty-free testing methods, and packaging that reduces waste and carbon footprint. Companies that can demonstrate their commitment to sustainability through certifications, eco-labels, and transparent supply chains are likely to gain a competitive advantage in the market. Ethical considerations extend to the social implications of nanotechnology, including the potential for unequal access to advanced cosmetic products. The premium pricing of many nano-cosmetics may create disparities in access, with these products being more readily available to higher-income consumers. Addressing these ethical concerns requires a balanced approach that ensures the benefits of nanotechnology are accessible to a broader population, without compromising safety or efficacy. Looking ahead, several trends are expected to shape the future of the nano-cosmetics industry. One of the most significant trends is the continued innovation in nanomaterial development, leading to the creation of new nanoparticles with enhanced properties and functions. This includes the development of stimuli-responsive nanoparticles that can release active ingredients in response to specific triggers, such as temperature or pH changes, offering even greater precision in targeted delivery [47]. Personalization will also be a key trend, with advances in nanotechnology enabling the customization of cosmetics based on individual genetic profiles, skin types, and environmental exposures. This level of personalization promises to deliver highly tailored skincare solutions, enhancing both the efficacy and consumer satisfaction of nano-cosmetics. Another emerging trend is the integration of nanotechnology with digital tools, such as skin analysis apps and smart beauty devices. These technologies can analyze skin conditions in real-time and recommend nano-cosmetics that are best suited to the user's needs, creating a seamless and personalized beauty experience [48]. Finally, the emphasis on sustainability and ethical production will continue to grow, with companies investing in green nanotechnology and developing biodegradable nanoparticles. The focus will be on reducing the environmental impact of nano-cosmetics throughout their lifecycle, from production to disposal, aligning with the broader industry movement towards sustainability and responsible innovation.

Table 2.2. Various nano-cosmetics available in the market.

Product Name	Brand	Nanomaterials Used	Claims/Benefits	Key Ingredients	Market Segment	References
L'Oréal Revitalift Laser X3	L'Oréal Paris	Pro-Xylane nanoparticles	Anti-aging, reduces wrinkles, and firms skin	Hyaluronic Acid, LHA	Anti-aging skincare	[49]
Olay Regenerist Micro-Sculpting Cream	Olay	Peptide nanoparticles	Skin firming, hydration, lifting effect	Amino-peptides, Hyaluronic Acid	Anti-aging skincare	[50]
Lancôme Génifique Youth Activating Concentrate	Lancôme	Biolysat nanoparticles	Anti-aging, boosts radiance, smooths fine lines	Probiotics, Bifidus extract	Anti-aging serum	[51]
Clinique Smart Custom-Repair Serum	Clinique	Liposomes	Targeted treatment, reduces wrinkles, and brightens	Peptides, Glucosamine	Skincare serum	[52]
Chanel Hydra Beauty Micro Sérum	Chanel	Camellia micro-droplets	Intense hydration, plumping effect	Camellia Alba PFA, Blue Ginger PFA	Hydrating serum	[53]
Estée Lauder Advanced Night Repair	Estée Lauder	Nano-emulsions	Anti-aging, hydration, and improves skin tone.	Hyaluronic Acid, ChronoluxCB™	Night serum	[54]

(Table 2.2) cont.....

Product Name	Brand	Nanomaterials Used	Claims/Benefits	Key Ingredients	Market Segment	References
Neutrogena Hydro Boost Water Gel	Neutrogena	Hyaluronic Acid nanoparticles	Hydration, skin elasticity	Hyaluronic Acid	Hydrating skincare	[55]
Shiseido Ultimune Power Infusing Concentrate	Shiseido	ImuGeneration Technology nanoparticles	Anti-aging, and strengthens skin's defenses	Reishi Mushroom, Iris Root Extract	Skincare booster	[56]
Vichy Minéral 89 Hyaluronic Acid Serum	Vichy	Hyaluronic Acid nanoparticles	Hydration, plumping, and strengthens the skin barrier.	Hyaluronic Acid, Vichy Volcanic Water	Hydrating skincare	[57]
Elizabeth Arden Prevage Anti-Aging Daily Serum	Elizabeth Arden	Idebenone nanoparticles	Anti-aging, environmental protection	Idebenone, Thiotaine	Anti-aging skincare	[58]
Garnier SkinActive Clearly Brighter	Garnier	Vitamin C nanoparticles	Brightens skin tone, and reduces dark spots.	Vitamin C, Antioxidants	Brightening skincare	[59]
Nanoblur Instant Skin Perfector	Indeed Labs	Nano-diffusing particles	Blurs imperfections, mattifies skin	Water, Glycerin	Instant skin perfector	[60]
La Roche-Posay Anthelios Mineral Sunscreen SPF 50	La Roche-Posay	Zinc Oxide nanoparticles	Broad-spectrum UV protection, sensitive skin	Zinc Oxide, and Titanium Dioxide	Sunscreen	[61]

CHALLENGES AND FUTURE DIRECTIONS

The field of nano-cosmetics, while brimming with potential, faces several significant challenges that must be addressed to fully realize its benefits. These challenges are not only technical but also encompass ethical and environmental concerns. Understanding these challenges and the prospects for innovation provides a comprehensive view of the current landscape and future direction of nano-cosmetics. The development of nano-cosmetics involves intricate technical challenges that stem from the complex nature of nanoparticles and their interactions with biological systems [62]. One of the foremost challenges is ensuring the stability of nanoparticles in cosmetic formulations. Nanoparticles are prone to agglomeration, where they clump together, losing their nano-scale properties and, consequently, their effectiveness. Ensuring that nanoparticles remain stable and evenly dispersed in cosmetic formulations over the product's shelf life requires sophisticated formulation techniques and stabilization agents.

Another significant technical challenge is controlling the penetration depth of nanoparticles into the skin. While deep skin penetration can be desirable for delivering active ingredients to specific layers of the skin, there is a risk of nanoparticles penetrating too deeply, potentially entering the bloodstream and causing unintended effects [63]. This requires precise control over the size, surface properties, and composition of nanoparticles to achieve the desired balance between efficacy and safety. The reproducibility and scalability of nano-cosmetic formulations pose technical challenges. Producing nanoparticles with consistent size, shape, and properties on a large scale, while maintaining the cost-effectiveness of the product, is a complex process that requires advanced manufacturing techniques and quality control measures. Variability in these parameters can lead to inconsistencies in product performance, which can affect consumer trust and satisfaction.

The rapid growth of the nano-cosmetics industry has sparked significant ethical and environmental concerns that must be carefully managed. One of the primary ethical concerns is the lack of comprehensive long-term studies on the safety of nanoparticles used in cosmetics. While many nanoparticles are considered safe for topical use, the long-term effects of chronic exposure, especially to nano-sized materials that can potentially penetrate the skin, are not fully understood. This uncertainty raises ethical questions about the responsibility of companies to ensure the safety of their products before widespread commercialization [64]. Environmental concerns are also paramount, particularly regarding the potential impact of nanoparticles on ecosystems. Once used, nano-cosmetic products are washed off and can enter waterways, where nanoparticles may interact with aquatic life. The small size and reactive nature of nanoparticles mean they can have unpredictable effects on marine organisms, potentially disrupting ecosystems and food chains. The persistence of nanoparticles in the environment and their potential to bioaccumulate further exacerbate these concerns [65]. The production and disposal of nano-cosmetics raise sustainability issues. The manufacturing processes for nanoparticles often involve hazardous chemicals and high energy consumption, which can contribute to environmental pollution and resource depletion. The disposal of nano-cosmetic products, particularly those with non-biodegradable nanoparticles, adds to the growing problem of microplastic pollution. These environmental challenges necessitate the development of green nanotechnology practices that minimize environmental impact and promote sustainability.

Despite these challenges, the future of nano-cosmetics is bright, with numerous prospects for innovation that promise to enhance the efficacy, safety, and sustainability of these products. One of the most promising areas of innovation is the development of smart nanoparticles, which can respond to environmental triggers such as temperature, pH, or light to release active ingredients precisely when and where they are needed [66]. This smart delivery system could significantly improve the performance of nano-cosmetics, offering targeted treatment with minimal waste of active ingredients. Advances in biomimetic nanotechnology, where nanoparticles mimic biological systems, also hold great potential for the future of nano-cosmetics. These bio-inspired nanoparticles can interact more effectively with the skin, enhancing absorption and minimizing adverse reactions. For example, lipid-based nanoparticles that mimic the natural lipid composition of the skin barrier could offer enhanced moisturization and protection [67]. Innovation in the formulation of eco-friendly nanoparticles is another promising direction. Researchers are exploring the use of natural and biodegradable materials to create nanoparticles that are less likely to persist in the environment. These sustainable nanoparticles could provide the same benefits as traditional nanoparticles while addressing environmental concerns. Personalized skincare powered by artificial intelligence (AI) and data analytics can recommend nano-cosmetic products tailored to individual skin types and conditions, enhancing their effectiveness and consumer satisfaction Additionally, smart packaging that can monitor product stability or track usage patterns could further enhance the consumer experience [68].

CONCLUSION

Nano-cosmetics have redefined skincare and beauty products by utilizing nanomaterials that enhance the delivery and performance of active ingredients, resulting in products that are not only more effective but also more appealing to consumers. The innovative formulations made possible by nanoparticles, nanoemulsions, liposomes, and niosomes have set new standards in the industry, offering solutions that address a wide range of consumer needs, from anti-aging to skin hydration and protection. The rapid growth and adoption of nano-cosmetics come with inherent challenges, particularly in ensuring the safety and regulatory compliance of these products. The potential risks associated with nanomaterials necessitate rigorous safety assessments and adherence to regulatory guidelines set forth by agencies like the FDA and EMA. As the industry continues to evolve, companies must prioritize consumer safety and transparency, fostering trust and confidence in nano-cosmetics. The chapter also highlights the changing landscape of the nano-cosmetics market, where consumer preferences are increasingly shaped by awareness of nanotechnology and its benefits. As consumers become more informed, their expectations for product performance, safety, and ethical considerations grow. This shift presents both opportunities and challenges for the industry, driving innovation while also demanding greater responsibility in product development and marketing.

REFERENCES

[1]   Mohanty, A.; Parida, A.; Raut, R.K.; Behera, R.K. Ferritin: A promising nanoreactor and nanocarrier for bionanotechnology. *ACS Bio & Med Chem Au,* **2022**, *2*(3), 258-281.
        [http://dx.doi.org/10.1021/acsbiomedchemau.2c00003] [PMID: 37101573]

[2]   Müller, R.H.; Radtke, M.; Wissing, S.A. Solid lipid nanoparticles (SLN) and nanostructured lipid carriers (NLC) in cosmetic and dermatological preparations. *Adv. Drug Deliv. Rev.,* **2002**, *54* Suppl. 1, S131-S155.
        [http://dx.doi.org/10.1016/S0169-409X(02)00118-7] [PMID: 12460720]

[3]   Jacobs, J.F.; van de Poel, I.; Osseweijer, P. Sunscreens with Titanium Dioxide (TiO_2) Nano-Particles: A Societal Experiment. *NanoEthics,* **2010**, *4*(2), 103-113.
        [http://dx.doi.org/10.1007/s11569-010-0090-y] [PMID: 20835397]

[4]   Patra, J.K.; Das, G.; Fraceto, L.F.; Campos, E.V.R.; Rodriguez-Torres, M.P.; Acosta-Torres, L.S.; Diaz-Torres, L.A.; Grillo, R.; Swamy, M.K.; Sharma, S.; Habtemariam, S.; Shin, H.S. Nano based drug delivery systems: recent developments and future prospects. *J. Nanobiotechnology,* **2018**, *16*(1), 71.
        [http://dx.doi.org/10.1186/s12951-018-0392-8] [PMID: 30231877]

[5]   Monteiro-Riviere, N.A.; Wiench, K.; Landsiedel, R.; Schulte, S.; Inman, A.O.; Riviere, J.E. Safety evaluation of sunscreen formulations containing titanium dioxide and zinc oxide nanoparticles in UVB sunburned skin: an *in vitro* and *in vivo* study. *Toxicol. Sci.,* **2011**, *123*(1), 264-280.
        [http://dx.doi.org/10.1093/toxsci/kfr148] [PMID: 21642632]

[6]   Kong, M.; Chen, X. Dong Keon Kweon; Do Hyun Park. *Investigations on Skin Permeation of Hyaluronic Acid Based Nanoemulsion as Transdermal Carrier.,* **2011**, *86*(2), 837-843.
        [http://dx.doi.org/10.1016/j.carbpol.2011.05.027]

[7]   Khan, I. Isoflavones-Based Liposome Formulations as Anti-Aging for Skincare. *Novel Approaches in Drug Designing & Development,* **2018**, *3*(3).
        [http://dx.doi.org/10.19080/NAPDD.2018.03.555615]

[8]   Fathi, M.; Mozafari, M.R.; Mohebbi, M. Nanoencapsulation of food ingredients using lipid based delivery systems. *Trends Food Sci. Technol.,* **2012**, *23*(1), 13-27.
        [http://dx.doi.org/10.1016/j.tifs.2011.08.003]

[9]   Mitchell, M.J.; Billingsley, M.M.; Haley, R.M.; Wechsler, M.E.; Peppas, N.A.; Langer, R. Engineering precision nanoparticles for drug delivery. *Nat. Rev. Drug Discov.,* **2021**, *20*(2), 101-124.
        [http://dx.doi.org/10.1038/s41573-020-0090-8] [PMID: 33277608]

[10]   Lohani, A.; Verma, A.; Joshi, H.; Yadav, N.; Karki, N. Nanotechnology-Based Cosmeceuticals. *ISRN Dermatol.,* **2014**, *2014*, 1-14.
        [http://dx.doi.org/10.1155/2014/843687] [PMID: 24963412]

[11]   Ganesan, P.; Choi, D.K. Current application of phytocompound-based nanocosmeceuticals for beauty and skin therapy. *Int. J. Nanomedicine,* **2016**, *2016*, 1987.
        [http://dx.doi.org/10.2147/IJN.S104701] [PMID: 27274231]

[12]   Rai, M.; Yadav, A.; Gade, A. Silver nanoparticles as a new generation of antimicrobials. *Biotechnol. Adv.,* **2009**, *27*(1), 76-83.
        [http://dx.doi.org/10.1016/j.biotechadv.2008.09.002] [PMID: 18854209]

[13]   Souto, E.B.; Fernandes, A.R.; Martins-Gomes, C.; Coutinho, T.E.; Durazzo, A.; Lucarini, M.; Souto, S.B.; Silva, A.M.; Santini, A. Nanomaterials for skin delivery of cosmeceuticals and pharmaceuticals. *Appl. Sci. (Basel),* **2020**, *10*(5), 1594.
        [http://dx.doi.org/10.3390/app10051594]

[14]   Tahir, R.; Albargi, H.B.; Ahmad, A.; Qadir, M.B.; Khaliq, Z.; Nazir, A.; Khalid, T.; Batool, M.; Arshad, S.N.; Jalalah, M.; Alsareii, S.A.; Harraz, F.A. Development of Sustainable Hydrophilic *Azadirachta indica* Loaded PVA Nanomembranes for Cosmetic Facemask Applications. *Membranes*

(Basel), **2023**, *13*(2), 156-156.
[http://dx.doi.org/10.3390/membranes13020156] [PMID: 36837659]

[15]   Jain, J.; Arora, S.; Rajwade, J.M.; Omray, P.; Khandelwal, S.; Paknikar, K.M. Silver nanoparticles in therapeutics: development of an antimicrobial gel formulation for topical use. *Mol. Pharm.*, **2009**, *6*(5), 1388-1401.
[http://dx.doi.org/10.1021/mp900056g] [PMID: 19473014]

[16]   Dhoundiyal, S.; Alam, M.A.; Kaur, A.; Sharma, S. Nanomedicines: Impactful approaches for targeting pulmonary diseases. *Pharm. Nanotechnol.*, **2024**, *12*(1), 14-31.
[http://dx.doi.org/10.2174/2211738511666230525151106] [PMID: 37231722]

[17]   Niroumand, H.; Zain, M.F.M.; Alhosseini, S.N. The Influence of Nano-clays on Compressive Strength of Earth Bricks as Sustainable Materials. *Procedia Soc. Behav. Sci.*, **2013**, *89*, 862-865.
[http://dx.doi.org/10.1016/j.sbspro.2013.08.945]

[18]   Fang, J.Y.; Fang, C.L.; Liu, C.H.; Su, Y.H. Lipid nanoparticles as vehicles for topical psoralen delivery: Solid lipid nanoparticles (SLN) *versus* nanostructured lipid carriers (NLC). *Eur. J. Pharm. Biopharm.*, **2008**, *70*(2), 633-640.
[http://dx.doi.org/10.1016/j.ejpb.2008.05.008] [PMID: 18577447]

[19]   McClements, D.J.; Rao, J. Food-grade nanoemulsions: formulation, fabrication, properties, performance, biological fate, and potential toxicity. *Crit. Rev. Food Sci. Nutr.*, **2011**, *51*(4), 285-330.
[http://dx.doi.org/10.1080/10408398.2011.559558] [PMID: 21432697]

[20]   Bravo, J.; Zhai, L.; Wu, Z.; Cohen, R.E.; Rubner, M.F. Transparent superhydrophobic films based on silica nanoparticles. *Langmuir*, **2007**, *23*(13), 7293-7298.
[http://dx.doi.org/10.1021/la070159q] [PMID: 17523683]

[21]   Alfadul, S.M.; Elneshwy, A.A. Use of nanotechnology in food processing, packaging and safety – review. *Afr. J. Food Agric. Nutr. Dev.*, **2010**, *10*(6).
[http://dx.doi.org/10.4314/ajfand.v10i6.58068]

[22]   Prabhu, S.; Poulose, E.K. Silver nanoparticles: mechanism of antimicrobial action, synthesis, medical applications, and toxicity effects. *Int. Nano Lett.*, **2012**, *2*(1), 32.
[http://dx.doi.org/10.1186/2228-5326-2-32]

[23]   Makadia, H.K.; Siegel, S.J. Poly Lactic-co-Glycolic Acid (PLGA) as Biodegradable Controlled Drug Delivery Carrier. *Polymers (Basel)*, **2011**, *3*(3), 1377-1397.
[http://dx.doi.org/10.3390/polym3031377] [PMID: 22577513]

[24]   Singh, R.; Lillard, J.W., Jr Nanoparticle-based targeted drug delivery. *Exp. Mol. Pathol.*, **2009**, *86*(3), 215-223.
[http://dx.doi.org/10.1016/j.yexmp.2008.12.004] [PMID: 19186176]

[25]   Jamkhande, P.G.; Ghule, N.W.; Bamer, A.H.; Kalaskar, M.G. Metal nanoparticles synthesis: An overview on methods of preparation, advantages and disadvantages, and applications. *J. Drug Deliv. Sci. Technol.*, **2019**, *53*, 101174.
[http://dx.doi.org/10.1016/j.jddst.2019.101174]

[26]   Yadwade, R.; Gharpure, S.; Ankamwar, B. Nanotechnology in cosmetics pros and cons. *Nano Express*, **2021**, *2*(2), 022003.
[http://dx.doi.org/10.1088/2632-959X/abf46b]

[27]   Antunes, A.F.; Pereira, P.; Reis, C.; Rijo, P.; Reis, C. Nanosystems for Skin Delivery: From Drugs to Cosmetics. *Curr. Drug Metab.*, **2017**, *18*(5), 412-425.
[http://dx.doi.org/10.2174/1389200218666170306103101] [PMID: 28266273]

[28]   Reza Mozafari, M.; Johnson, C.; Hatziantoniou, S.; Demetzos, C. Nanoliposomes and their applications in food nanotechnology. *J. Liposome Res.*, **2008**, *18*(4), 309-327.
[http://dx.doi.org/10.1080/08982100802465941] [PMID: 18951288]

[29]   Choy, J.; Choi, S.; Oh, J.; Park, T. Clay minerals and layered double hydroxides for novel biological

applications. *Appl. Clay Sci.,* **2007**, *36*(1-3), 122-132.
[http://dx.doi.org/10.1016/j.clay.2006.07.007]

[30] Bilal, M.; Iqbal, H.M.N. New insights on unique features and role of nanostructured materials in cosmetics. *Cosmetics,* **2020**, *7*(2), 24.
[http://dx.doi.org/10.3390/cosmetics7020024]

[31] Müller, R.; Petersen, R.; Hommoss, A.; Pardeike, J. Nanostructured lipid carriers (NLC) in cosmetic dermal products. *Adv. Drug Deliv. Rev.,* **2007**, *59*(6), 522-530.
[http://dx.doi.org/10.1016/j.addr.2007.04.012] [PMID: 17602783]

[32] Alves, T.F.R.; Morsink, M.; Batain, F.; Chaud, M.V.; Almeida, T.; Fernandes, D.A.; da Silva, C.F.; Souto, E.B.; Severino, P. Applications of natural, semi-synthetic, and synthetic polymers in cosmetic formulations. *Cosmetics,* **2020**, *7*(4), 75.
[http://dx.doi.org/10.3390/cosmetics7040075]

[33] Hirsch, L.R.; Stafford, R.J.; Bankson, J.A.; Sershen, S.R.; Rivera, B.; Price, R.E.; Hazle, J.D.; Halas, N.J.; West, J.L. Nanoshell-mediated near-infrared thermal therapy of tumors under magnetic resonance guidance. *Proc. Natl. Acad. Sci. USA,* **2003**, *100*(23), 13549-13554.
[http://dx.doi.org/10.1073/pnas.2232479100] [PMID: 14597719]

[34] Nel, A.; Xia, T.; Mädler, L.; Li, N. Toxic potential of materials at the nanolevel. *Science,* **2006**, *311*(5761), 622-627.
[http://dx.doi.org/10.1126/science.1114397] [PMID: 16456071]

[35] Connor, E.E.; Mwamuka, J.; Gole, A.; Murphy, C.J.; Wyatt, M.D. Gold nanoparticles are taken up by human cells but do not cause acute cytotoxicity. *Small,* **2005**, *1*(3), 325-327.
[http://dx.doi.org/10.1002/smll.200400093] [PMID: 17193451]

[36] He, H.; Li, A.; Li, S.; Tang, J.; Li, L.; Xiong, L., Natural components in sunscreens: Topical formulations with sun protection factor (SPF). *Biomed. Pharmacother.,* **2021**, *134*, 111161.
[http://dx.doi.org/10.1016/j.biopha.2020.111161]

[37] Peters, R.; Brandhoff, P.; Weigel, S.; Marvin, H.; Bouwmeester, H.; Aschberger, K.; Rauscher, H.; Amenta, V.; Arena, M.; Botelho Moniz, F.; Gottardo, S.; Mech, A. Inventory of Nanotechnology applications in the agricultural, feed and food sector. *EFSA Support. Publ.,* **2014**, *11*(7).
[http://dx.doi.org/10.2903/sp.efsa.2014.EN-621]

[38] Turner, B. *International Organization for Standardization*; ISO, **2003**, pp. 47-47.

[39] Ray, P.C.; Yu, H.; Fu, P.P. Toxicity and environmental risks of n: Challenges and future needs. *J. Environ. Sci. Health Part C Environ. Carcinog. Ecotoxicol. Rev.,* **2009**, *27*(1), 1-35.
[http://dx.doi.org/10.1080/10590500802708267]

[40] Amberg, N.; Fogarassy, C. Green Consumer Behavior in the Cosmetics Market. *Resources,* **2019**, *8*(3), 137.
[http://dx.doi.org/10.3390/resources8030137]

[41] Lodén, M. Role of topical emollients and moisturizers in the treatment of dry skin barrier disorders. *Am. J. Clin. Dermatol.,* **2003**, *4*(11), 771-788.
[http://dx.doi.org/10.2165/00128071-200304110-00005] [PMID: 14572299]

[42] Hemantha, L.M.I.T.; Gayathri, T.M.E.; Silva, N.N.M.D. Personalized Smart Skincare Product Recommendation System. *Int. J. Comput. Appl.,* **2022**, *184*(41), 1-6.
[http://dx.doi.org/10.5120/ijca2022922469]

[43] Shevchenko, R.V.; James, S.L.; James, S.E. A review of tissue-engineered skin bioconstructs available for skin reconstruction. *J. R. Soc. Interface,* **2010**, *7*(43), 229-258.
[http://dx.doi.org/10.1098/rsif.2009.0403] [PMID: 19864266]

[44] Stuart, M.A.C.; Huck, W.T.S.; Genzer, J.; Müller, M.; Ober, C.; Stamm, M.; Sukhorukov, G.B.; Szleifer, I.; Tsukruk, V.V.; Urban, M.; Winnik, F.; Zauscher, S.; Luzinov, I.; Minko, S. Emerging applications of stimuli-responsive polymer materials. *Nat. Mater.,* **2010**, *9*(2), 101-113.

[http://dx.doi.org/10.1038/nmat2614] [PMID: 20094081]

[45] Iavicoli, I.; Leso, V.; Fontana, L.; Bergamaschi, A. Toxicological effects of titanium dioxide nanoparticles: a review of *in vitro* mammalian studies. *Eur. Rev. Med. Pharmacol. Sci.*, **2011**, *15*(5), 481-508.
[PMID: 21744743]

[46] Pei, Y.; Wang, L.; Tang, K.; Kaplan, D.L. Biopolymer nanoscale assemblies as building blocks for new materials: A review. *Adv. Funct. Mater.*, **2021**, *31*(15), 2008552.
[http://dx.doi.org/10.1002/adfm.202008552]

[47] Zha, L.; Banik, B.; Alexis, F. Stimulus responsive nanogels for drug delivery. *Soft Matter,* **2011**, *7*(13), 5908.
[http://dx.doi.org/10.1039/c0sm01307b]

[48] Frigaard, J.; Jensen, J.L.; Galtung, H.K.; Hiorth, M. The Potential of Chitosan in Nanomedicine: An Overview of the Cytotoxicity of Chitosan Based Nanoparticles. *Front. Pharmacol.*, **2022**, *13*, 880377.
[http://dx.doi.org/10.3389/fphar.2022.880377] [PMID: 35600854]

[49] Bouloc, A.; Roo, E.; Moga, A.; Chadoutaud, B.; Zouboulis, C. A compensating skin care complex containing pro-xylane in menopausal women: results from a multicentre, evaluator-blinded, randomized study. *Acta Derm. Venereol.*, **2017**, *97*(4), 541-542.
[http://dx.doi.org/10.2340/00015555-2572] [PMID: 27840889]

[50] Ahsan, H. The significance of complex polysaccharides in personal care formulations. *J. Carbohydr. Chem.*, **2019**, *38*(4), 213-233.
[http://dx.doi.org/10.1080/07328303.2019.1615498]

[51] Talebi, E.; Haghighat Jahromi, M. Effect of Olive Leaves Hydroalcoholic Extract (*Olea Europaea* L.) and LactoFeed® probiotics on Induced Ascites in Male Broilers. *Tekirdag Ziraat Fak. Derg.*, **2023**, *20*(3), 688-697.
[http://dx.doi.org/10.33462/jotaf.1250068]

[52] Rabasco Alvarez, A.M.; González Rodríguez, M.L. Lipids in pharmaceutical and cosmetic preparations. *Grasas Aceites,* **2000**, *51*(1-2), 74-96.
[http://dx.doi.org/10.3989/gya.2000.v51.i1-2.409]

[53] Searing, C.; Zeilig, H. Fine Lines: cosmetic advertising and the perception of ageing female beauty. *Int. J. Ageing Later Life,* **2017**, *11*(1), 7-36.
[http://dx.doi.org/10.3384/ijal.1652-8670.16-290]

[54] Zhong, Y. Indicator Analysis for Cosmetics Companies: Evidence from L'Oréal, Shiseido and Estée Lauder. *Highlights in Business, Economics and Management*, **2023**, *7*, 42-46.
[http://dx.doi.org/10.54097/hbem.v7i.6824]

[55] Al-Qadi, S.; Alatorre-Meda, M.; Zaghloul, E.M.; Taboada, P.; Remunán-López, C. Chitosan–hyaluronic acid nanoparticles for gene silencing: The role of hyaluronic acid on the nanoparticles' formation and activity. *Colloids Surf. B Biointerfaces,* **2013**, *103*, 615-623.
[http://dx.doi.org/10.1016/j.colsurfb.2012.11.009] [PMID: 23274155]

[56] Jiang, B.; Jia, Y.; He, C. Promoting new concepts of skincare *via* skinomics and systems biology—From traditional skincare and efficacy-based skincare to precision skincare. *J. Cosmet. Dermatol.*, **2018**, *17*(6), 968-976.
[http://dx.doi.org/10.1111/jocd.12663] [PMID: 29749695]

[57] Nemitz, M.C.; Moraes, R.C.; Koester, L.S.; Bassani, V.L.; von Poser, G.L.; Teixeira, H.F. Bioactive soy isoflavones: extraction and purification procedures, potential dermal use and nanotechnology-based delivery systems. *Phytochem. Rev.*, **2015**, *14*(5), 849-869.
[http://dx.doi.org/10.1007/s11101-014-9382-0]

[58] Rashid, J. Muhammad Farooq Sabar; Gill, Z.; Mustafa, U.; Fatima, S.; Ashiq, S. Cosmeceuticals: The bioactive elements in new-age beauty products. *International Journal of Pharmacy & Integrated*

Health Sciences, **2023**, *4*(2), 70-82.
[http://dx.doi.org/10.56536/ijpihs.v4i2.98]

[59]   Teng, Z.; Luo, Y.; Wang, Q. Carboxymethyl chitosan–soy protein complex nanoparticles for the encapsulation and controlled release of vitamin D3. *Food Chem.,* **2013**, *141*(1), 524-532.
[http://dx.doi.org/10.1016/j.foodchem.2013.03.043] [PMID: 23768389]

[60]   Seddiqi, H.; Oliaei, E.; Honarkar, H.; Jin, J.; Geonzon, L.C.; Bacabac, R.G.; Klein-Nulend, J. Cellulose and its derivatives: towards biomedical applications. *Cellulose,* **2021**, *28*(4), 1893-1931.
[http://dx.doi.org/10.1007/s10570-020-03674-w]

[61]   Bidart, P. *La Roche-Posay. ADLFI*; Archéologie de la France - Informations, **2009**.
[http://dx.doi.org/10.4000/adlfi.3286]

[62]   Development and Stability Evaluation of Liquid Crystal-Based Formulations Containing Glycolic Plant Extracts and Nano-Actives. *Cosmetics,* **2018**, *5*(2), 25.
[http://dx.doi.org/10.3390/cosmetics5020025]

[63]   Prausnitz, M.R.; Langer, R. Transdermal drug delivery. *Nat. Biotechnol.,* **2008**, *26*(11), 1261-1268.
[http://dx.doi.org/10.1038/nbt.1504] [PMID: 18997767]

[64]   Far, J.; Abdel-Haq, M.; Gruber, M.; Abu Ammar, A. Developing Biodegradable Nanoparticles Loaded with Mometasone Furoate for Potential Nasal Drug Delivery. *ACS Omega,* **2020**, *5*(13), 7432-7439.
[http://dx.doi.org/10.1021/acsomega.0c00111] [PMID: 32280885]

[65]   Limbach, L.K.; Bereiter, R.; Müller, E.; Krebs, R.; Gälli, R.; Stark, W.J. Removal of oxide nanoparticles in a model wastewater treatment plant: influence of agglomeration and surfactants on clearing efficiency. *Environ. Sci. Technol.,* **2008**, *42*(15), 5828-5833.
[http://dx.doi.org/10.1021/es800091f] [PMID: 18754516]

[66]   Hood, E. Nanotechnology: looking as we leap. *Environ. Health Perspect.,* **2004**, *112*(13), A740-A749.
[http://dx.doi.org/10.1289/ehp.112-a740] [PMID: 15345364]

[67]   Wang, Z.; Wang, Z.; Lu, W.W.; Zhen, W.; Yang, D.; Peng, S. Novel biomaterial strategies for controlled growth factor delivery for biomedical applications. *NPG Asia Mater.,* **2017**, *9*(10), e435-e435.
[http://dx.doi.org/10.1038/am.2017.171]

[68]   C, A.; R, D.K. IoT-Enabled Skincare Devices for Personalized Beauty and Wellness. *International Journal of Research Publication and Reviews,* **2024**, *5*(3), 389-393.
[http://dx.doi.org/10.55248/gengpi.5.0324.0611]

CHAPTER 3

Nanotechnology in Textiles and Wearables

Abstract: In this chapter, we discuss the integration of nanotechnology in textiles and wearables, highlighting its transformative impact on the industry. It begins with an overview of nanotechnology in the textile sector, exploring its significance and historical evolution. The concept of smart fabrics and functional clothing is then introduced, detailing the types of nanomaterials used, including conductive nanomaterials, nano-coatings, and nanocomposites. Applications such as temperature-regulating clothing, self-cleaning fabrics, and garments with embedded sensors are examined. The discussion extends to wearable health monitors, focusing on the role of nanotechnology in enhancing these devices, particularly through nanostructured sensors and nano-biosensors. The chapter also covers the integration of AI and data analytics in health monitors and the commercial landscape, addressing key industry players, successful case studies, and the impact on fashion and sportswear. Finally, it explores regulatory, ethical, environmental, and sustainability considerations, concluding with insights into future trends and opportunities in this rapidly evolving field.

Keywords: Artificial Intelligence, Industry, Nano coatings, Textiles, Wearables.

INTRODUCTION

Nanotechnology, which involves the manipulation and control of matter at the nanoscale, has significantly transformed the textile industry. At this scale, materials exhibit unique physical and chemical properties, enabling the formation of textiles with enhanced strength, durability, and elasticity. Incorporating nanoparticles such as carbon nanotubes into textiles can greatly improve their tensile strength without adding extra weight [1]. Additionally, nanotechnology allows for the application of nano-coatings that impart various functional finishes to fabrics, including water repellency, stain resistance, UV protection, and antimicrobial effects. These coatings are often invisible to the naked eye, preserving the fabric's original texture and appearance [2]. Nanofibers, created through processes like electrospinning, produce highly porous and lightweight fabrics that can be engineered for specific functionalities, such as filtration or thermal insulation. Nano-composites, which embed nanoparticles within a matrix material, offer enhanced mechanical and thermal properties, opening up new possibilities for textiles that meet both aesthetic and comfort requirements while providing additional functionalities [3]. This shows that the role of nanotechnology in the textile industry has enabled the development of specialized fabrics for applications in sports, medicine, military, and everyday use. Wearable technology, which includes electronic devices or components worn on the body, has also benefited immensely from nanotechnology. The miniaturization enabled by nanotechnology is critical for creating wearable devices that are comfortable and non-intrusive. Nanostructured sensors, for example, can detect and monitor a wide range of physiological parameters, such as heart rate, body temperature, and glucose levels, with greater sensitivity and accuracy than larger sensors [4]. This makes them ideal for continuous health monitoring. Nanotechnology also plays a crucial role in energy harvesting and storage for wearable devices. Flexible and lightweight energy storage devices, like supercapacitors and batteries, can be integrated into wearable textiles, while nanomaterials in energy harvesting systems convert body movements or environmental energy into electrical energy to power these devices. Additionally, nanotechnology allows for the development of flexible and breathable materials that are comfortable to wear over extended periods. The ability to produce transparent or nearly invisible electronic components ensures that the aesthetic appeal of wearable clothing is maintained. The applications of nanotechnology in wearable technology are diverse, ranging from fitness trackers and health monitors to smart clothing that can adapt to environmental conditions [5]. This integration is driving the evolution of wearables from simple gadgets to multifunctional tools that enhance users' health, safety, and quality of life. Although a relatively recent development, the application of nanotechnology in textiles and wearables has deep roots in the history of materials science and electronics. Historically, the concept of enhancing textiles with advanced materials is not new. For centuries, humans have sought to improve fabric properties through various methods, such as chemical treatments and blending fibers. However, it was not until the late 20th century that the idea of using nanoscale materials became feasible. The term "nanotechnology" was popularized by physicist Richard Feynman in the 1950s, but significant advancements in microscopy and fabrication techniques in the 1980s and 1990s allowed scientists to manipulate materials at the nanoscale. The textile industry quickly recognized the potential of these technologies for improving fabric performance and introducing new functionalities. By the early 2000s, the first commercial applications of nanotechnology in textiles began to appear, including wrinkle-resistant and stain-repellent clothing, as well as fabrics with enhanced durability [6]. Companies experimented with nano-coatings and embedded nanoparticles to create textiles with superior properties. The convergence of nanotechnology and wearable electronics gained momentum in the late 2000s and early 2010s, driven by the growing demand for portable and connected devices. Innovations such as flexible displays, nanowire sensors, and conductive fabrics enabled the development of wearable devices that were not only functional but also discreet and comfortable to wear. In recent years, there has been a surge in the development of smart fabrics and wearables with integrated health monitoring capabilities. Advances in nanomaterials, such as graphene and other 2D materials, have further expanded the possibilities, leading to the creation of fabrics that can monitor vital signs, detect environmental hazards, and even generate energy [7]. The historical development of nanotechnology in textiles and wearables is marked by a series of innovations that have progressively enhanced the capabilities of fabrics and wearable devices, making them an integral part of modern life.

SMART FABRICS AND FUNCTIONAL CLOTHING

Smart fabrics, also known as e-textiles or intelligent textiles, are materials that have been engineered to sense and respond to external stimuli or environmental changes. Unlike traditional fabrics, which serve primarily aesthetic and protective functions, smart fabrics are imbued with advanced functionalities through the integration of electronic components, sensors, and nanomaterials. These fabrics can detect changes in temperature, pressure, humidity, and other environmental factors, and then react accordingly. For example, some smart fabrics can adjust their thermal properties to regulate the wearer's body temperature or change color in response to UV exposure, as depicted in Fig. (**3.1**) [8]. The characteristics of smart fabrics include flexibility, durability, and the ability to seamlessly integrate with electronic components without compromising the fabric's comfort or appearance. These fabrics are often designed to be lightweight and breathable, ensuring they can be worn comfortably for extended periods. Smart fabrics are typically washable and resistant to wear and tear, crucial for their practical use in everyday clothing [9]. The development of smart fabrics represents a significant advancement in textile technology, offering new possibilities for applications in fashion, healthcare, sports, and military fields, where combining traditional textile properties with cutting-edge technology can provide enhanced functionality and user experience.

Types of Nanomaterials used in Smart Fabrics

Conductive nanomaterials play a critical role in the development of smart fabrics by enabling the integration of electronic functionality into textiles. These materials are engineered at the nanoscale to conduct electricity while maintaining the fabric's flexibility and comfort. Common conductive nanomaterials used in smart fabrics include silver nanowires, carbon nanotubes, and graphene. Silver nanowires are highly conductive and can be woven or printed onto fabrics to create electrical pathways, making them ideal for applications such as wearable sensors, heating elements, and even touch-sensitive surfaces [10]. Carbon nanotubes, with their excellent electrical conductivity and mechanical strength, are often used in smart fabrics that require flexible and stretchable electronics. Graphene, a single layer of carbon atoms arranged in a hexagonal lattice, is celebrated for its extraordinary electrical conductivity and thinness, allowing it to be used in fabrics without adding bulk [11]. These conductive nanomaterials enable smart fabrics to interact with electronic devices, transmit data, and respond to external stimuli, paving the way for innovative applications in wearable technology, healthcare monitoring, and interactive clothing.

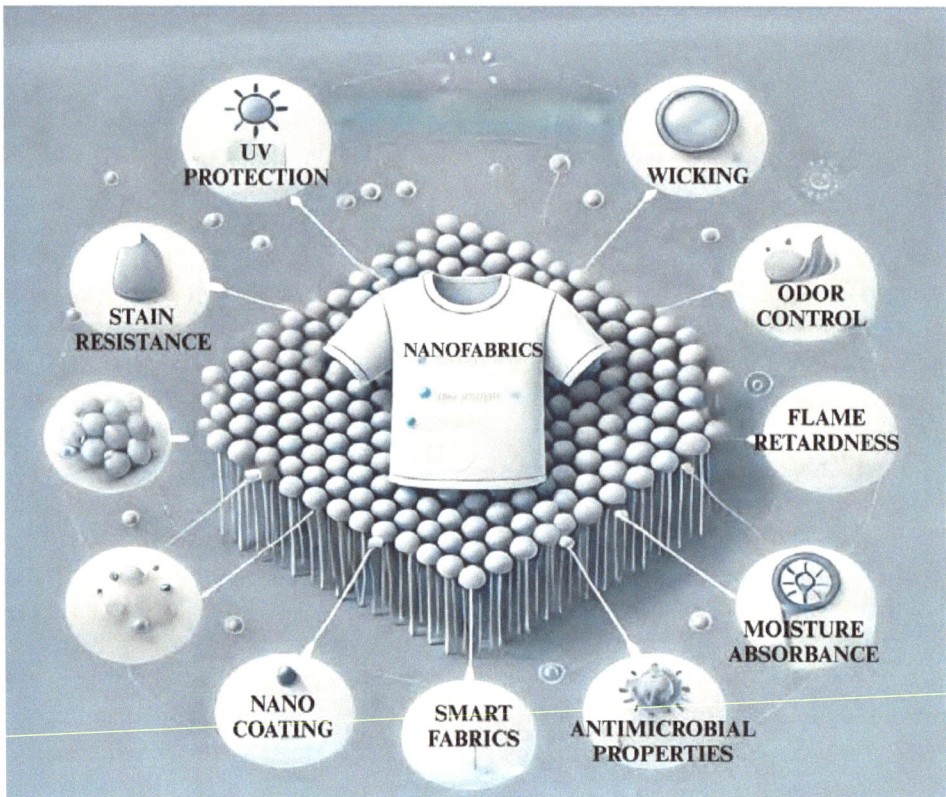

Fig. (3.1). Application of nano-based fabrics.

Nano-coatings are thin layers of nanomaterials applied to the surface of textiles to impart additional functionalities without altering the fabric's inherent properties. These coatings can provide a range of benefits, including water repellency, stain resistance, UV protection, and antimicrobial properties. For example, hydrophobic nano-coatings, often made from nanoparticles like silica or titanium dioxide, create a water-repellent surface that prevents liquids from soaking into the fabric, making the textiles easier to clean and maintain [12]. Similarly, nano-coatings infused with silver or copper nanoparticles can impart antimicrobial properties, reducing the growth of bacteria and odors in the fabric, which is particularly useful in medical textiles and activewear. Additionally, nano-coatings can enhance the durability of textiles by protecting them from wear and tear, as well as environmental degradation [13]. These coatings are typically invisible and do not affect the fabric's feel, ensuring that the comfort and appearance of the clothing are preserved while adding new functional layers to the textile.

Nanocomposites are materials that combine nanoparticles with a matrix, such as polymers, to create fabrics that are both durable and flexible. These composites are designed to enhance the mechanical properties of textiles, making them stronger, more resistant to damage, and better suited for demanding applications. Nanoparticles such as carbon nanotubes, nanoclays, and metal oxides are commonly used in these composites to reinforce the fabric, providing increased tensile strength, toughness, and abrasion resistance [14]. The flexibility of nanocomposites allows them to be used in smart fabrics that need to withstand repeated bending, stretching, and folding without losing their structural integrity. This is particularly important for wearable technology, where comfort and durability are paramount. Nanocomposites can also be engineered to provide additional functionalities, such as thermal regulation or electromagnetic shielding, making them versatile materials for various smart fabric applications. By using these advanced nanomaterials, smart fabrics can achieve a balance of strength, flexibility, and enhanced performance, expanding their potential uses in both consumer and industrial markets.

Applications of Smart Fabrics

Temperature-regulating clothing is an innovative application of smart fabrics designed to maintain the wearer's comfort by adjusting to changes in environmental or body temperature. These fabrics often incorporate phase change materials (PCMs) at the nanoscale, which absorb, store, and release heat as they transition between solid and liquid states [15]. When the body temperature rises, the PCMs absorb excess heat, providing a cooling effect, and when the body temperature drops, the stored heat is released to warm the wearer. This dynamic thermal management ensures that the clothing adapts to the wearer's needs, enhancing comfort in varying weather conditions. Additionally, conductive nanomaterials can be used in temperature-regulating clothing to distribute heat evenly across the fabric, preventing hot or cold spots. Such clothing is particularly beneficial for outdoor activities, sports, and environments where temperature fluctuations are common. By applying these advanced materials, temperature-regulating smart fabrics offer both functionality and comfort, making them a significant advancement in wearable technology [16].

Self-cleaning and anti-microbial fabrics are another key application of smart fabrics, providing enhanced hygiene and convenience for the wearer. These fabrics are treated with nano-coatings or embedded with nanoparticles, such as titanium dioxide, silver, or zinc oxide, which have self-cleaning and antimicrobial properties. Titanium dioxide, for example, is a photocatalyst that, when exposed to sunlight, breaks down organic matter and contaminants on the fabric surface, effectively cleaning the fabric without the need for washing [17]. Silver nanoparticles, known for their antimicrobial properties, inhibit the growth of bacteria, fungi, and other microorganisms, reducing odors and the risk of infections. These properties are particularly valuable in medical textiles, activewear, and garments worn in environments where hygiene is crucial. Self-cleaning fabrics not only reduce the frequency of laundering but also extend the lifespan of the clothing by preventing stains and wear caused by frequent washing. By incorporating these nanomaterials, smart fabrics provide a practical solution to maintaining cleanliness and hygiene, making them highly desirable in both consumer and industrial applications.

Sensing and actuating garments represent a sophisticated application of smart fabrics, integrating sensors and actuators within the textile to monitor and respond to various stimuli [18]. These garments are embedded with nanosensors that can detect physiological parameters such as heart rate, respiration, body temperature, and movement. The data collected by these sensors can be used for health monitoring, fitness tracking, or even to provide real-time feedback during physical activities. Actuators, on the other hand, enable the garment to perform actions in response to the sensed data. For instance, a jacket embedded with actuators might tighten or loosen depending on the wearer's body temperature or posture, or a pair of gloves might vibrate to alert the wearer of an incoming message [19]. These garments are particularly valuable in healthcare, where continuous monitoring of vital signs can provide early detection of health issues, and in sports, where they can enhance performance through precise feedback. The use of sensing and actuating capabilities in smart fabrics transforms ordinary clothing into interactive, multifunctional devices that enhance the user experience in various settings.

Integration of Electronics in Smart Fabrics

Sensors embedded within the fabric are designed to detect a wide range of physiological and environmental parameters, such as temperature, humidity, pressure, and motion. These sensors are often made from nanomaterials like carbon nanotubes, silver nanowires, or graphene, which provide high sensitivity while being lightweight and flexible enough to be woven or printed into textiles. For instance, heart rate sensors embedded in a fitness shirt can monitor the wearer's cardiovascular activity in real-time, transmitting data to a connected device for analysis [20]. Similarly, pressure sensors in smart shoes can track gait and foot pressure, providing valuable data for improving posture or preventing injuries.

Actuators, on the other hand, enable the fabric to respond to the data collected by the sensors. These responses can range from simple actions, such as changing the color of the fabric in response to light exposure, to more complex behaviors like adjusting the tightness of a garment or activating vibration motors in response to specific movements or signals. For example, a smart jacket might include actuators that tighten around the waist when the temperature drops, providing additional warmth, or release tension during physical activity to enhance comfort [21]. The integration of sensors and actuators transforms textiles into interactive systems that not only monitor the wearer's environment but also provide immediate feedback or adjustments, enhancing both functionality and user experience. Power supply and energy harvesting are crucial elements for the functionality of smart fabrics, as these garments require a reliable source of energy to operate their embedded electronics [22]. Traditional batteries, though effective, can add bulk and weight to smart textiles, potentially compromising comfort and wearability. To address this challenge, researchers and developers are increasingly turning to flexible, lightweight, and even wearable power solutions. One approach involves the use of thin, flexible batteries or supercapacitors that can be integrated directly into the fabric or garment structure. These power sources are designed to be bendable and conform to the shape of the body, ensuring they do not interfere with the fabric's natural movement or the wearer's comfort [23].

Energy harvesting is another innovative solution for powering smart fabrics. This technology involves capturing energy from the wearer's movements, body heat, or even environmental sources like sunlight and converting it into electrical power. For instance, piezoelectric materials embedded in the fabric can generate electricity when the fabric is stretched or compressed during movement [24]. Similarly, thermoelectric generators can convert the temperature difference between the body and the external environment into usable energy. Solar panels made from flexible photovoltaic materials can be incorporated into outdoor garments to capture solar energy, providing a sustainable power source for wearable electronics. These advancements in power supply and energy harvesting are essential for the continued development of smart fabrics, enabling more sophisticated applications and broader adoption in everyday life.

WEARABLE HEALTH MONITORS

Wearable health technologies are revolutionizing the way individuals monitor and manage their health by providing real-time access to vital health data. These devices, which include smartwatches, fitness trackers, and smart clothing, are designed to be worn continuously, allowing for constant monitoring of physiological parameters such as heart rate, blood pressure, glucose levels, and physical activity, as illustrated in Fig. (**3.2**) [25]. The data collected by these devices can be synced with smartphones or other digital platforms, enabling users to track their health trends, set fitness goals, and even receive alerts about potential health issues. The rise of wearable health monitors is driven by advances in sensor technology, miniaturization of electronic components, and the increasing demand for personalized healthcare solutions. These technologies not only empower individuals to take proactive control of their health but also provide valuable data that can be shared with healthcare providers for more informed decision-making. As wearable health monitors become more sophisticated, they are increasingly being used in clinical settings to monitor patients with chronic conditions, support rehabilitation, and even detect early signs of disease. The role of artificial intelligence (AI) and machine learning in these devices further enhances their capabilities, allowing for more accurate data interpretation and personalized health recommendations [26]. As a result, wearable health technologies are becoming an essential tool in modern healthcare, offering users both convenience and advanced health insights. Energy harvesting is another innovative solution for powering smart fabrics. This technology involves capturing energy from the wearer's movements, body heat, or even environmental sources like sunlight and converting it into electrical power. Piezoelectric materials embedded in the fabric can generate electricity when the fabric is stretched or compressed during movement [27]. Similarly, thermoelectric generators can convert the temperature difference between the body and the external environment into usable energy. Solar panels made from flexible photovoltaic materials can be incorporated into outdoor garments to capture solar energy, providing a sustainable power source for wearable electronics [28]. Smart fabrics can become more self-sufficient, reducing the need for external power sources and enhancing the practicality and longevity of wearable devices. These advancements in power supply and energy harvesting are essential for the continued development of smart fabrics, enabling more sophisticated applications and broader adoption in everyday life.

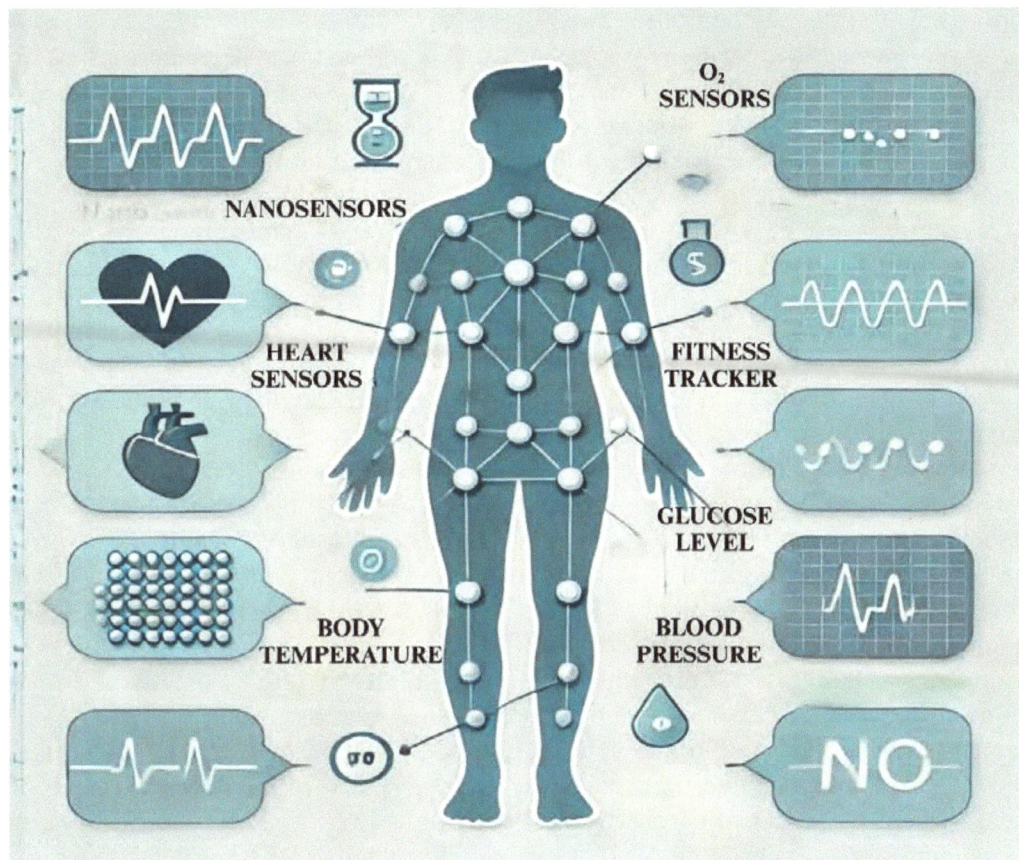

Fig. (3.2). Nano based sensors for monitoring health.

Nanotechnology in Health Monitoring Devices

Nanostructured sensors are at the forefront of advancements in health monitoring devices, offering unprecedented sensitivity and accuracy in tracking vital signs. These sensors are designed to detect minute changes in physiological parameters such as the heart rate, respiratory rate, body temperature, and blood pressure. The high surface area-to-volume ratio of nanomaterials, such as carbon nanotubes, graphene, and gold nanoparticles, enables them to interact more effectively with biological molecules, leading to faster and more precise measurements. For instance, wearable devices equipped with nanostructured sensors can continuously monitor a patient's heart rate with high fidelity, providing real-time data that can alert users or healthcare providers to abnormal conditions, such as arrhythmias or sudden changes in the heart rate [29].

The nanostructured sensors in wearable devices also enhance their usability and comfort, as these sensors can be embedded into flexible, lightweight materials that conform to the body's contours. This allows for continuous monitoring without the discomfort associated with bulkier traditional devices. Furthermore, the miniaturization of these sensors means they can be incorporated into a wide range of wearable formats, from wristbands and patches to smart textiles, making them versatile tools in both personal health management and clinical settings [30]. As these technologies evolve, nanostructured sensors are likely to play an increasingly critical role in the early detection and management of health conditions, offering users a seamless way to monitor their vital signs and maintain their well-being.

Nano-biosensors represent a significant advancement in the field of health monitoring, particularly for the detection and management of biomarkers like glucose. These biosensors utilize nanomaterials to detect the presence of specific biological molecules at extremely low concentrations, enabling precise monitoring of biomarkers that are critical for managing conditions such as diabetes. For glucose monitoring, nano-biosensors are often integrated into wearable devices that provide continuous, non-invasive glucose readings [31]. This is achieved through the use of nanostructured materials like gold nanoparticles or carbon nanotubes, which interact with glucose molecules in bodily fluids, such as sweat or interstitial fluid, and generate an electrical signal proportional to the glucose concentration. Beyond glucose, nano-biosensors are being developed to monitor a variety of other biomarkers, including lactate, cholesterol, and even specific proteins or hormones that indicate the presence of diseases such as cancer or cardiovascular conditions [32]. The high sensitivity and specificity of these sensors make them valuable tools for early diagnosis and real-time health monitoring. Additionally, the data collected by these nano-biosensors can be transmitted to connected devices, allowing for continuous tracking and analysis, which is essential for personalized medicine and tailored healthcare interventions. As the technology progresses, nano-biosensors are expected to become more integrated into everyday health monitoring devices, providing users with comprehensive insights into their health and enabling proactive management of chronic conditions.

Types of Wearable Health Monitors

Fitness trackers are among the most common and widely used types of wearable health monitors, designed to track and analyze a range of physical activities and vital signs. These devices typically come in the form of wristbands or smartwatches and are equipped with sensors that monitor metrics such as steps taken, calories burned, distance travelled, and heart rate. More advanced models also track sleep patterns, blood oxygen levels, and even stress levels by measuring heart rate variability [33]. Fitness trackers are popular for their ability to provide real-time feedback, helping users set and achieve fitness goals, monitor their progress, and make informed decisions about their health and lifestyle. The data collected by fitness trackers can be synced with mobile apps or cloud-based platforms, allowing users to analyze trends over time and share their progress with others. Many fitness trackers also offer features like reminders to move, guided breathing exercises, and notifications for reaching specific activity milestones. These devices cater to a broad audience, from casual users looking to maintain an active lifestyle to athletes seeking detailed performance insights [34]. The convenience and accessibility of fitness trackers have made them an essential tool for anyone looking to integrate health monitoring into their daily routine. Continuous health monitoring systems represent a more advanced category of wearable health monitors, designed for the ongoing tracking of critical health parameters in real-time. These systems are particularly valuable for individuals with chronic health conditions, such as diabetes, hypertension, or cardiovascular diseases, who require regular monitoring to manage their health effectively. Continuous health monitoring devices are often integrated with sensors that measure vital signs like heart rate, blood pressure, glucose levels, and oxygen saturation [35]. Unlike fitness trackers, these systems are designed for medical-grade accuracy and often provide data that can be shared directly with healthcare providers for remote monitoring and management.

One of the key benefits of continuous health monitoring systems is their ability to detect and alert users to potential health issues before they become critical, allowing for timely intervention. For instance, continuous glucose monitors (CGMs) are widely used by individuals with diabetes to monitor glucose levels throughout the day and night, providing alerts for hyperglycemia or hypoglycemia [36]. Similarly, wearable ECG monitors can track heart activity continuously, detecting arrhythmias or other cardiac events in real-time. These systems often include data analytics and AI-driven insights to help users and healthcare professionals make informed decisions based on the collected data, making them a cornerstone of personalized and preventive healthcare. Wearable therapeutic devices are a specialized type of wearable health monitors that not only track health data but also provide therapeutic interventions [37]. These devices are designed to treat or manage specific health conditions through targeted therapies, often using technologies such as electrical stimulation, drug delivery, or thermal regulation. For example, wearable devices that provide transcutaneous electrical nerve stimulation (TENS) can help relieve chronic pain by delivering small electrical impulses to nerve endings. Other therapeutic wearables include insulin pumps for diabetes management, which continuously deliver insulin to the body based on real-time glucose readings from a connected monitor [38]. In addition to these, wearable therapeutic devices are being developed for applications such as rehabilitation, where they can assist in physical therapy by guiding and monitoring exercises, or for mental health, where they may provide biofeedback or neurostimulation to help manage conditions like anxiety or depression. These devices offer the advantage of continuous, at-home therapy, reducing the need for frequent visits to healthcare facilities and allowing for more personalized and adaptive treatment plans. By combining monitoring and therapeutic functions, wearable therapeutic devices represent a significant advancement in the field of digital health, providing both immediate relief and long-term management of health conditions.

Commercial Applications

The market for wearable health monitors has seen a rapid expansion, driven by innovations in technology and a growing demand for health-focused devices. Commercial products in this space range from simple fitness trackers to advanced medical-grade monitors that offer continuous health tracking, as mentioned in Table **3.1**. Brands like Fitbit, Apple, Garmin, and Samsung dominate the consumer market, offering devices that integrate multiple health metrics such as heart rate, sleep patterns, and activity levels into a single wearable device [39]. These products often come equipped with user-friendly interfaces, mobile app integration, and the ability to sync data across multiple platforms, making health monitoring accessible to a broad audience. In addition to consumer-grade products, there has been a surge in specialized devices designed for clinical and professional use. These include wearable ECG monitors, continuous glucose monitors (CGMs), and devices that monitor respiratory function, all of which are being used to manage chronic diseases and monitor patients remotely. Innovations in this sector are continually pushing the boundaries, with advancements in nanotechnology, flexible electronics, and AI-driven analytics contributing to the development of more sophisticated and accurate monitoring solutions. Wearable health monitors are also increasingly incorporating features such as real-time feedback, personalized health recommendations, and emergency alerts, making them indispensable tools for both personal health management and professional healthcare [40]. The wearable health monitor industry is highly competitive, with several major players leading the charge in innovation and market share. Companies like Apple, Fitbit (now part of Google), and Samsung have established themselves as leaders in the consumer wearable market, with products like the Apple Watch and Fitbit series becoming household names. These companies are known for their focus on integrating health monitoring features into everyday devices, making them attractive to a wide range of consumers. Apple, in particular, has made significant strides in incorporating advanced health features such as ECG monitoring, blood oxygen measurement, and even fall detection into its Apple Watch, positioning it as a leader in health-focused wearables. In the medical-grade wearables sector, companies like Medtronic, Dexcom, and Abbott are at the forefront, particularly in the development of continuous glucose monitors and other specialized health monitoring devices [41]. These companies are focused on providing accurate, reliable, and FDA-approved devices that are used in clinical settings and for chronic disease management. The industry is also seeing the emergence of new players and startups, particularly in the realm of AI-driven health analytics and personalized health monitoring solutions. These companies are leveraging cutting-edge technology to develop wearables that not only track health metrics but also provide actionable insights and personalized care recommendations. The combination of established industry giants and innovative newcomers is driving the wearable health monitor market towards greater sophistication and broader adoption.

Table 3.1. Commercial applications of nanotechnology in textiles and wearables.

Category	Application	Description	Examples/Products	References
Smart Fabrics	**Temperature-Regulating Clothing**	Utilizes phase-change materials and thermoregulatory nanomaterials to maintain optimal body temperature.	Outlast® technology, ThermalTech jackets	[45
-	**Self-Cleaning and Anti-Microbial Fabrics**	Incorporates nano-coatings or silver nanoparticles that repel dirt and eliminate bacteria, keeping fabrics clean and hygienic.	NanoSphere® by Schoeller, NanoHorizons' SmartSilver®	[46, 47]
-	**Sensing and Actuating Garments**	Embeds sensors and actuators to monitor body movements, vital signs, and environmental conditions, enabling real-time feedback and interaction.	Hexoskin Smart Shirts, Sensoria Fitness Socks	[48]
-	**UV-Protection Clothing**	Uses nanoparticles like titanium dioxide or zinc oxide to block harmful UV rays, protecting the wearer from sun damage.	SunSoul clothing, Coolibar's UV-protective wear	[49]
-	**Stain-Resistant and Water-Repellent Fabrics**	Nanotechnology is applied to create fabrics that resist staining and water absorption, enhancing durability and usability.	Nano-Tex®, NeverWet® by Rust-Oleum	[50]

(Table 3.1) cont.....

Category	Application	Description	Examples/Products	References
-	**Fire-Resistant Fabrics**	Utilizes nanocoatings to improve flame retardancy, providing enhanced safety for industrial and protective clothing.	Teijin's Aramid Nanofiber Technology	[51]
Wearable Health Monitors	**Fitness Trackers**	Devices embedded in fabrics or worn as accessories that monitor physical activity, heart rate, sleep patterns, and more.	Fitbit, Apple Watch	[52]
-	**Continuous Health Monitoring Systems**	Advanced wearables that continuously monitor vital signs like blood pressure, glucose levels, and provide real-time health data to users.	FreeStyle Libre, BioIntelliSense BioButton	[53]
-	**Wearable Therapeutic Devices**	Wearables that deliver therapies, such as drug delivery or pain management, based on monitored health data.	Quell Relief, Omron HeartGuide	[54]
-	**Wearable Safety Monitors**	Used in industrial and hazardous environments to monitor exposure to toxins, gas levels, and environmental conditions.	Blackline Safety G7, Honeywell's wearable gas detectors	[55]
-	**Smart Eyewear and Headsets**	Integrates AR, VR, and health monitoring features in eyewear, providing data overlays, and health insights directly to the user.	Google Glass Enterprise Edition, Vuzix M400 Smart Glasses	[56]
Impact on Fashion and Sportswear	**High-Performance Sportswear**	Nanotechnology-enhanced fabrics that offer moisture-wicking, cooling, and enhanced comfort features for athletes and active wear.	Under Armour ColdGear®, Nike Dri-FIT	[57]
-	**Smart Accessories**	Accessories like belts, gloves, and hats embedded with sensors for monitoring health, providing security, or enhancing user interaction.	Levi's Commuter x Jacquard by Google, Oura Ring	[58]

(Table 3.1) cont.....

Category	Application	Description	Examples/Products	References
-	**Wearable Displays**	Clothing or accessories with embedded screens or displays, allowing for personalized messages or visual effects controlled by the user.	Luminex by CuteCircuit, Twinkling Stars Shirt by Komatsu	[59]

Case studies of successful wearable health products provide insight into the factors that contribute to their widespread adoption and impact on the market. The Apple Watch, for instance, is a prime example of a product that has successfully integrated advanced health monitoring features with everyday functionality [42]. Since its introduction, the Apple Watch has evolved from a fitness-focused device to a comprehensive health monitoring tool, offering features such as ECG monitoring, blood oxygen levels, and sleep tracking. Its success can be attributed to Apple's ability to blend seamless user experience with powerful health features, as well as its strong brand loyalty and integration with the broader Apple ecosystem. Another successful case is the Fitbit series, which pioneered the concept of wearable fitness tracking and has maintained a strong market presence through continuous innovation and expansion into health monitoring. Fitbit's devices are known for their accuracy in tracking physical activity, heart rate, and sleep patterns, and the company has successfully leveraged its large user base and data-driven insights to refine its products over time. Fitbit's acquisition by Google has further positioned it to integrate with broader health data systems and expand its capabilities. In the medical wearables category, Dexcom's continuous glucose monitors (CGMs) are a standout example of a product that has transformed diabetes management. Dexcom's CGMs provide real-time glucose readings, which can be monitored remotely by patients and healthcare providers [43]. The success of these devices lies in their ability to provide accurate, continuous data, reduce the need for finger-prick tests, and enhance the quality of life for individuals with diabetes. These case studies highlight the importance of innovation, user experience, and the ability to meet specific health needs in the success of wearable health products.

The role of wearable health monitors in fashion and sportswear has significantly impacted these industries, leading to the emergence of smart textiles and functional clothing that combine style with advanced health monitoring capabilities. In the fashion industry, there has been a growing trend towards incorporating wearable technology into everyday apparel, making health monitoring a seamless part of daily life. Designers and technology companies are collaborating to create clothing that can track physiological parameters while maintaining aesthetic appeal. For example, smart jackets, shirts, and even accessories like rings and bracelets are being developed with embedded sensors that monitor vital signs, stress levels, and even UV exposure. In the sportswear industry, wearable health monitors are revolutionizing how athletes and fitness enthusiasts train and manage their health [44]. Brands like Nike, Under Armour, and Adidas are integrating sensor technology into their apparel and footwear to track performance metrics such as speed, distance, heart rate, and muscle activity. These innovations provide athletes with real-time feedback and data analytics to optimize their training regimes and prevent injuries. The fusion of health monitoring with sportswear has also led to the development of specialized products such as compression garments with embedded sensors for muscle recovery and smart shoes that track running form. The impact of wearable health monitors on fashion and sportswear industries extends beyond just product innovation; it also influences consumer behavior and expectations. As these technologies become more integrated into clothing and accessories, consumers are increasingly seeking products that offer both functionality and style. This shift is driving the fashion and sportswear industries to adopt more technology-driven approaches, creating new opportunities for innovation and growth.

CHALLENGES

The rise of wearable health monitors brings forth significant regulatory and ethical considerations that must be addressed to ensure their safe and responsible use. Regulatory bodies like the U.S. Food and Drug Administration (FDA) and the European Medicines Agency (EMA) are increasingly involved in overseeing the development and approval of these devices, especially those intended for medical use. Wearable health monitors that claim to diagnose, treat, or manage medical conditions are subject to rigorous testing and validation to ensure their accuracy, reliability, and safety [60]. This regulatory oversight is crucial to prevent the distribution of devices that could provide misleading health information, which could lead to misdiagnosis or improper treatment. Ethical considerations also play a critical role in the development and deployment of wearable health monitors. Issues such as data privacy, consent, and the potential for misuse of health data are at the forefront of these concerns. As these devices collect sensitive health information, there is a growing need to ensure that this data is stored securely and used ethically. Users must be fully informed about how their data will be used and who will have access to it [61]. Additionally, there is the question of equity in access to these technologies. Ensuring that wearable health monitors are accessible and affordable to a broad population, rather than just a privileged few, is essential for their ethical deployment. The potential for these devices to be used in employer or insurance contexts raises concerns about discrimination or surveillance based on health data. Addressing these ethical challenges requires ongoing dialogue among technology developers, regulators, ethicists, and the public to establish clear guidelines and protections that uphold individual rights and societal values.

The proliferation of wearable health monitors also raises important environmental and sustainability issues that must be addressed to minimize their ecological impact. The production and disposal of electronic devices, including wearables, contribute to e-waste, which is a growing environmental concern. Many wearable devices contain non-biodegradable materials and hazardous substances such as heavy metals, which can be harmful if not disposed of properly [62]. As the demand for wearable technology increases, so does the need for sustainable practices in their design, manufacturing, and end-of-life management. To address these challenges, companies are increasingly focusing on developing eco-friendly wearables that incorporate sustainable materials and are designed for longevity. This includes using recycled materials, reducing the use of toxic substances, and designing products that are easier to repair or recycle. For example, some companies are exploring the use of biodegradable polymers and organic electronics that have a lower environmental footprint. Additionally, efforts are being made to develop energy-efficient wearables that require less power and have longer battery life, reducing the frequency of charging and the environmental impact associated with battery production and disposal. Another key aspect of sustainability is the push towards circular economy models, where wearable devices are designed with modular components that can be easily replaced or upgraded, extending the device's lifespan and reducing waste [63]. Companies are also implementing take-back programs to ensure that used devices are recycled or disposed of responsibly. As awareness of environmental issues grows, the development of sustainable wearable health monitors is likely to become a priority, with consumers increasingly demanding products that are not only technologically advanced but also environmentally responsible.

FUTURE DIRECTIONS

The future of wearable health monitors is poised to be shaped by several exciting trends and opportunities that promise to revolutionize healthcare and personal wellness. One of the most significant trends is the integration of artificial intelligence and machine learning into wearable devices. AI-powered wearables can analyze vast amounts of health data in real-time, providing users with personalized insights and predictive analytics. This can help in the early detection of health issues, personalized treatment plans, and more informed decision-making, both for individuals and healthcare providers [64]. Another emerging trend is the development of more advanced and multifunctional wearables that go beyond simple health tracking. These devices are expected to incorporate features such as continuous non-invasive monitoring of glucose, hydration levels, or even biomarkers for stress and fatigue. The integration of flexible and stretchable electronics will allow these wearables to be seamlessly embedded into clothing and other textiles, making them more comfortable and unobtrusive. Additionally, advancements in energy harvesting technologies, such as solar cells and kinetic energy converters, are expected to power wearables without the need for frequent charging, enhancing their usability and convenience. The convergence of wearables with other technologies, such as augmented reality (AR) and virtual reality (VR), is also anticipated to open up new opportunities in areas like remote diagnostics, telemedicine, and rehabilitation. For example, AR glasses with embedded health monitoring sensors could provide real-time data overlays during physical activities or medical consultations, enhancing the user's experience and providing valuable health insights [65]. The growing focus on holistic health and wellness is likely to drive the development of wearables that monitor not just physical health but also mental and emotional well-being. These could include devices that track biomarkers associated with stress, anxiety, or sleep quality, offering users tools to manage their mental health more effectively. As these trends unfold, the wearable health monitor market is expected to see significant growth, driven by technological advancements, increasing consumer awareness, and the rising demand for personalized healthcare solutions. The continued evolution of this field holds the promise of more integrated, intelligent, and sustainable wearable technologies that will play a pivotal role in shaping the future of healthcare and wellness.

CONCLUSION

Nanotechnology has revolutionized the textiles and wearables industry, offering unprecedented opportunities for innovation and functionality. This chapter has explored how nanotechnology is being leveraged to create smart fabrics that not only enhance comfort and performance but also provide health-monitoring capabilities through integrated electronics. The discussion highlighted the diverse applications of these technologies, from temperature regulation and self-cleaning fabrics to advanced wearable health monitors that track vital signs and biomarkers. As the market for these technologies expands, driven by consumer demand and technological advancements, the importance of addressing regulatory, ethical, and environmental challenges becomes paramount. The chapter underscores the need for sustainable practices and responsible innovation to ensure that these technologies contribute positively to society. Looking ahead, the integration of AI, data analytics, and energy harvesting technologies in wearables promises to further advance the field, making personalized health monitoring and smart textiles an integral part of everyday life.

REFERENCES

[1]   Shi, P.; Li, L.; Hua, L.; Qian, Q.; Wang, P.; Zhou, J.; Sun, G.; Huang, W. Design of amorphous manganese oxide@multiwalled carbon nanotube fiber for robust solid-state supercapacitor. *ACS Nano,* **2017,** *11*(1), 444-452.
[http://dx.doi.org/10.1021/acsnano.6b06357] [PMID: 28027441]

[2]   Oberdörster, E. Manufactured nanomaterials (fullerenes, C60) induce oxidative stress in the brain of juvenile largemouth bass. *Environ. Health Perspect.,* **2004,** *112*(10), 1058-1062.
[http://dx.doi.org/10.1289/ehp.7021] [PMID: 15238277]

[3]   Incorporating Optimization to Improve Durability of A356 metal matrix composites with nanoparticles of TiO₂ and SiC. *Nanotechnol. Percept.,* **2024,** *20*(S1).
[http://dx.doi.org/10.62441/nano-ntp.v20iS1.11]

[4]   Chudzik, A.; Śledzianowski, A.; Przybyszewski, A.W. Machine learning and digital biomarkers can detect early stages of neurodegenerative diseases. *Sensors (Basel),* **2024,** *24*(5), 1572.
[http://dx.doi.org/10.3390/s24051572] [PMID: 38475108]

[5]   Zhu, C.; Wu, J.; Yan, J.; Liu, X. Advanced Fiber Materials for Wearable Electronics. *Advanced Fiber Materials,* **2023,** *5*(1), 12-35.
[http://dx.doi.org/10.1007/s42765-022-00212-0]

[6]   Khan, I.; Saeed, K.; Khan, I. Nanoparticles: Properties, applications and toxicities. *Arab. J. Chem.,* **2019,** *12*(7), 908-931.
[http://dx.doi.org/10.1016/j.arabjc.2017.05.011]

[7]   Lin, Y.; Ren, J.; Qu, X. Catalytically active nanomaterials: a promising candidate for artificial enzymes. *Acc. Chem. Res.,* **2014,** *47*(4), 1097-1105.
[http://dx.doi.org/10.1021/ar400250z] [PMID: 24437921]

[8]   Tao, X. Study of Fiber-Based Wearable Energy Systems. *Acc. Chem. Res.,* **2019,** *52*(2), 307-315.
[http://dx.doi.org/10.1021/acs.accounts.8b00502] [PMID: 30698417]

[9]   Xiong, J.; Lin, M.F.; Wang, J.; Gaw, S.L.; Parida, K.; Lee, P.S. Wearable All-Fabric-Based Triboelectric Generator for Water Energy Harvesting. *Adv. Energy Mater.,* **2017,** *7*(21), 1701243.
[http://dx.doi.org/10.1002/aenm.201701243]

[10]   Lee, S.; Shin, S.; Lee, S.; Seo, J.; Lee, J.; Son, S.; Cho, H.J.; Algadi, H.; Al-Sayari, S.; Kim, D.E.; Lee, T. Ag Nanowire Reinforced Highly Stretchable Conductive Fibers for Wearable Electronics. *Adv. Funct. Mater.,* **2015,** *25*(21), 3114-3121.
[http://dx.doi.org/10.1002/adfm.201500628]

[11]   Sanchez, V.C.; Jachak, A.; Hurt, R.H.; Kane, A.B. Biological interactions of graphene-family nanomaterials: an interdisciplinary review. *Chem. Res. Toxicol.,* **2012,** *25*(1), 15-34.
[http://dx.doi.org/10.1021/tx200339h] [PMID: 21954945]

[12]   Wu, W.; He, Q.; Jiang, C. Magnetic iron oxide nanoparticles: synthesis and surface functionalization strategies. *Nanoscale Res. Lett.,* **2008,** *3*(11), 397-415.
[http://dx.doi.org/10.1007/s11671-008-9174-9] [PMID: 21749733]

[13]   Rai, M.; Yadav, A.; Gade, A. Silver nanoparticles as a new generation of antimicrobials. *Biotechnol. Adv.,* **2009,** *27*(1), 76-83.
[http://dx.doi.org/10.1016/j.biotechadv.2008.09.002] [PMID: 18854209]

[14]   Kolya, H.; Kang, C.W. Next-Generation Water Treatment: Exploring the Potential of Biopolymer-Based Nanocomposites in Adsorption and Membrane Filtration. *Polymers (Basel),* **2023,** *15*(16), 3421.
[http://dx.doi.org/10.3390/polym15163421] [PMID: 37631480]

[15]   Mondal, S. Phase change materials for smart textiles – An overview. *Appl. Therm. Eng.,* **2008,** *28*(11-12), 1536-1550.
[http://dx.doi.org/10.1016/j.applthermaleng.2007.08.009]

[16]   Xu, J.; Wang, M.; Wickramaratne, N.P.; Jaroniec, M.; Dou, S.; Dai, L. High-performance sodium ion batteries based on a 3D anode from nitrogen-doped graphene foams. *Adv. Mater.,* **2015**, *27*(12), 2042-2048.
[http://dx.doi.org/10.1002/adma.201405370] [PMID: 25689053]

[17]   Sang, N.X.; Huong, P.T.L.; Thy, T.T.M.; Dat, P.T.; Minh, V.C.; Tho, N.H. Crystalline deformation and photoluminescence of titanium dioxide nanotubes during in situ hybridization with graphene: An example of the heterogeneous photocatalyst. *Superlattices Microstruct.,* **2018**, *121*, 9-15.
[http://dx.doi.org/10.1016/j.spmi.2018.07.020]

[18]   Awano, M.; Sando, M.; Niihara, K. Synthesis of Nanocomposite Ceramics for Magnetic Remote Sensing and Actuating. *Key Eng. Mater.,* **1998**, *161-163*, 485-488.
[http://dx.doi.org/10.4028/www.scientific.net/KEM.161-163.485]

[19]   Sarif Ullah Patwary, M.S. Smart Textiles and Nano-Technology: A General Overview. *J. Text. Sci. Eng.,* **2015**, *5*(1).
[http://dx.doi.org/10.4172/2165-8064.1000181]

[20]   Pantelopoulos, A.; Bourbakis, N.G. A Survey on Wearable Sensor-Based Systems for Health Monitoring and Prognosis. *IEEE Trans. Syst. Man Cybern. C,* **2010**, *40*(1), 1-12.
[http://dx.doi.org/10.1109/TSMCC.2009.2032660]

[21]   Design of Smart Cooling Jacket for 2-Wheeler Riders. *International Journal of Recent Trends in Engineering and Research,* **2018**, *4*(3), 211-216.
[http://dx.doi.org/10.23883/IJRTER.2018.4118.I7BH3]

[22]   Gungor, V.C.; Hancke, G.P. Industrial Wireless Sensor Networks: Challenges, Design Principles, and Technical Approaches. *IEEE Trans. Ind. Electron.,* **2009**, *56*(10), 4258-4265.
[http://dx.doi.org/10.1109/TIE.2009.2015754]

[23]   Pushparaj, V.L.; Shaijumon, M.M.; Kumar, A.; Murugesan, S.; Ci, L.; Vajtai, R.; Linhardt, R.J.; Nalamasu, O.; Ajayan, P.M. Flexible energy storage devices based on nanocomposite paper. *Proc. Natl. Acad. Sci. USA,* **2007**, *104*(34), 13574-13577.
[http://dx.doi.org/10.1073/pnas.0706508104] [PMID: 17699622]

[24]   Rus, D.; Tolley, M.T. Design, fabrication and control of soft robots. *Nature,* **2015**, *521*(7553), 467-475.
[http://dx.doi.org/10.1038/nature14543] [PMID: 26017446]

[25]   Walsh, J.A., III; Topol, E.J.; Steinhubl, S.R. Novel wireless devices for cardiac monitoring. *Circulation,* **2014**, *130*(7), 573-581.
[http://dx.doi.org/10.1161/CIRCULATIONAHA.114.009024] [PMID: 25114186]

[26]   Boon, I.S.; Au Yong, T.P.T.; Boon, C.S. Assessing the Role of Artificial Intelligence (AI) in Clinical Oncology: Utility of Machine Learning in Radiotherapy Target Volume Delineation. *Medicines (Basel),* **2018**, *5*(4), 131.
[http://dx.doi.org/10.3390/medicines5040131] [PMID: 30544901]

[27]   Rus, D.; Tolley, M.T. Design, fabrication and control of soft robots. *Nature,* **2015**, *521*(7553), 467-475.
[http://dx.doi.org/10.1038/nature14543] [PMID: 26017446]

[28]   Dallaev, R.; Pisarenko, T.; Papež, N.; Holcman, V. Overview of the Current State of Flexible Solar Panels and Photovoltaic Materials. *Materials (Basel),* **2023**, *16*(17), 5839-5839.
[http://dx.doi.org/10.3390/ma16175839] [PMID: 37687532]

[29]   Dunn, B.; Kamath, H.; Tarascon, J.M. Electrical energy storage for the grid: a battery of choices. *Science,* **2011**, *334*(6058), 928-935.
[http://dx.doi.org/10.1126/science.1212741] [PMID: 22096188]

[30]   Bonato, P. Advances in wearable technology and applications in physical medicine and rehabilitation. *J. Neuroeng. Rehabil.,* **2005**, *2*(1), 2.

[http://dx.doi.org/10.1186/1743-0003-2-2] [PMID: 15733322]

[31] Naresh, V.; Lee, N. A Review on Biosensors and Recent Development of Nanostructured Materials-Enabled Biosensors. *Sensors (Basel),* **2021**, *21*(4), 1109.
[http://dx.doi.org/10.3390/s21041109] [PMID: 33562639]

[32] Choi, W.; Choudhary, N.; Han, G.H.; Park, J.; Akinwande, D.; Lee, Y.H. Recent development of two-dimensional transition metal dichalcogenides and their applications. *Mater. Today,* **2017**, *20*(3), 116-130.
[http://dx.doi.org/10.1016/j.mattod.2016.10.002]

[33] Khayat, R.; Chaudhari, A.; Lee, E.; Kim, J. Utilizing novel sensor to track transient blood pressure changes during sleep. *Sleep Med.,* **2024**, *115*, S400.
[http://dx.doi.org/10.1016/j.sleep.2023.11.1077]

[34] Alderson, A. Sports Tech: Fitness Trackers. *Engineering & Technology,* **2015**, *10*(4), 84-85.
[http://dx.doi.org/10.1049/et.2015.0461]

[35] Evans, J.; Papadopoulos, A.; Silvers, C.T.; Charness, N.; Boot, W.R.; Schlachta-Fairchild, L.; Crump, C.; Martinez, M.; Ent, C.B. Remote health monitoring for older adults and those with heart failure: Adherence and system usability. *Telemed. J. E Health,* **2016**, *22*(6), 480-488.
[http://dx.doi.org/10.1089/tmj.2015.0140] [PMID: 26540369]

[36] Krinsley, J.S.; Chase, J.G.; Gunst, J.; Martensson, J.; Schultz, M.J.; Taccone, F.S.; Wernerman, J.; Bohe, J.; De Block, C.; Desaive, T.; Kalfon, P.; Preiser, J.C. Continuous glucose monitoring in the ICU: clinical considerations and consensus. *Crit. Care,* **2017**, *21*(1), 197.
[http://dx.doi.org/10.1186/s13054-017-1784-0] [PMID: 28756769]

[37] Arabian, H.; Abdulbaki Alshirbaji, T.; Schmid, R.; Wagner-Hartl, V.; Chase, J.G.; Moeller, K. Harnessing Wearable Devices for Emotional Intelligence: Therapeutic Applications in Digital Health. *Sensors (Basel),* **2023**, *23*(19), 8092-8092.
[http://dx.doi.org/10.3390/s23198092] [PMID: 37836923]

[38] Bergenstal, R.M.; Tamborlane, W.V.; Ahmann, A.; Buse, J.B.; Dailey, G.; Davis, S.N.; Joyce, C.; Peoples, T.; Perkins, B.A.; Welsh, J.B.; Willi, S.M.; Wood, M.A. Effectiveness of sensor-augmented insulin-pump therapy in type 1 diabetes. *N. Engl. J. Med.,* **2010**, *363*(4), 311-320.
[http://dx.doi.org/10.1056/NEJMoa1002853] [PMID: 20587585]

[39] Lee, I.; Shin, Y.J. Fintech: Ecosystem, business models, investment decisions, and challenges. *Bus. Horiz.,* **2018**, *61*(1), 35-46.
[http://dx.doi.org/10.1016/j.bushor.2017.09.003]

[40] Abbasi, J. Skin-like Wearable Health Monitors. *JAMA,* **2017**, *318*(14), 1314.
[http://dx.doi.org/10.1001/jama.2017.14440] [PMID: 29049568]

[41] Wagner, V.; Dullaart, A.; Bock, A.K.; Zweck, A. The emerging nanomedicine landscape. *Nat. Biotechnol.,* **2006**, *24*(10), 1211-1217.
[http://dx.doi.org/10.1038/nbt1006-1211] [PMID: 17033654]

[42] Gent, E. News: Apple iPhone6 and Apple Watch finally unveiled. *Engineering & Technology,* **2014**, *9*(9), 12-12.
[http://dx.doi.org/10.1049/et.2014.0904]

[43] Lal, R.A.; Maahs, D.M. Clinical Use of Continuous Glucose Monitoring in Pediatrics. *Diabetes Technol. Ther.,* **2017**, *19*(S2), S-37-S-43.
[http://dx.doi.org/10.1089/dia.2017.0013] [PMID: 28541138]

[44] Anwar, S.; Hassanpour Amiri, M.; Jiang, S.; Abolhasani, M.M.; Rocha, P.R.F.; Asadi, K. Piezoelectric Nylon-11 Fibers for Electronic Textiles, Energy Harvesting and Sensing. *Adv. Funct. Mater.,* **2021**, *31*(4), 2004326.
[http://dx.doi.org/10.1002/adfm.202004326]

[45] Tong, J.K.; Huang, X.; Boriskina, S.V.; Loomis, J.; Xu, Y.; Chen, G. Infrared-Transparent Visible-

Opaque Fabrics for Wearable Personal Thermal Management. *ACS Photonics,* **2015**, *2*(6), 769-778.
[http://dx.doi.org/10.1021/acsphotonics.5b00140]

[46]   Wong, H.; Yucn, M.; Leung, S.; Ku, A.; Lam, I. Selected applications of nanotechnology in textiles.
       AUTEX Research Journal. AUTEX Res. J., **2006**, *6*(1), 1-8.
       [http://dx.doi.org/10.1515/aut-2006-060101]

[47]   Yuan Gao, ; Cranston, R. Recent Advances in Antimicrobial Treatments of Textiles. *Text. Res. J.,*
       2008, *78*(1), 60-72.
       [http://dx.doi.org/10.1177/0040517507082332]

[48]   Angelucci, A.; Cavicchioli, M.; Cintorrino, I.; Lauricella, G.; Rossi, C.; Strati, S.; Aliverti, A. Smart
       Textiles and Sensorized Garments for Physiological Monitoring: A Review of Available Solutions and
       Techniques. *Sensors (Basel),* **2021**, *21*(3), 814.
       [http://dx.doi.org/10.3390/s21030814] [PMID: 33530403]

[49]   Barrow, M.M. Approaching skin cancer education with a clear message. *J. Dermatol. Nurses Assoc.,*
       2010, *2*(5), 209-213.
       [http://dx.doi.org/10.1097/JDN.0b013e3181f50cf0]

[50]   Shillingford, C.; MacCallum, N.; Wong, T.S.; Kim, P.; Aizenberg, J. Fabrics coated with lubricated
       nanostructures display robust omniphobicity. *Nanotechnology,* **2014**, *25*(1), 014019.
       [http://dx.doi.org/10.1088/0957-4484/25/1/014019] [PMID: 24334333]

[51]   Luo, J.; Zhang, M.; Yang, B.; Liu, G.; Tan, J.; Nie, J.; Song, S. A promising transparent and UV-
       shielding composite film prepared by aramid nanofibers and nanofibrillated cellulose. *Carbohydr.
       Polym.,* **2019**, *203*, 110-118.
       [http://dx.doi.org/10.1016/j.carbpol.2018.09.040] [PMID: 30318194]

[52]   Bai, Y.; Tompkins, C.; Gell, N.; Dione, D.; Zhang, T.; Byun, W. Comprehensive comparison of Apple
       Watch and Fitbit monitors in a free-living setting. *PLoS One,* **2021**, *16*(5), e0251975.
       [http://dx.doi.org/10.1371/journal.pone.0251975] [PMID: 34038458]

[53]   Yoo, J.; Yan, L.; Lee, S.; Kim, Y.; Yoo, H.J. A 5.2 mW Self-Configured Wearable Body Sensor
       Network Controller and a 12 $$W Wirelessly Powered Sensor for a Continuous Health Monitoring
       System. *IEEE J. Solid-State Circuits,* **2010**, *45*(1), 178-188.
       [http://dx.doi.org/10.1109/JSSC.2009.2034440]

[54]   Angelova, R.A. High-Performance Apparel and Wearable Devices for Hot Environments.
       International Journal of Mobile Devices, Wearable Technology, and Flexible Electronics, **2019**, *10*(1),
       1-14.
       [http://dx.doi.org/10.4018/IJMDWTFE.2019010101]

[55]   Awolusi, I.; Marks, E.; Hallowell, M. Wearable technology for personalized construction safety
       monitoring and trending: Review of applicable devices. *Autom. Construct.,* **2018**, *85*, 96-106.
       [http://dx.doi.org/10.1016/j.autcon.2017.10.010]

[56]   Kress, B.; Saeedi, E.; Brac-de-la-Perriere, V. The Segmentation of the HMD Market: Optics for Smart
       Glasses, Smart Eyewear, AR and vr Headsets. *Proc. SPIE,* **2014**, 92020D.
       [http://dx.doi.org/10.1117/12.2064351]

[57]   Farah, S.; Anderson, D.G.; Langer, R. Physical and mechanical properties of PLA, and their functions
       in widespread applications — A comprehensive review. *Adv. Drug Deliv. Rev.,* **2016**, *107*, 367-392.
       [http://dx.doi.org/10.1016/j.addr.2016.06.012] [PMID: 27356150]

[58]   Seneviratne, S.; Hu, Y.; Nguyen, T.; Lan, G.; Khalifa, S.; Thilakarathna, K.; Hassan, M.; Seneviratne,
       A. A Survey of Wearable Devices and Challenges. *IEEE Commun. Surv. Tutor.,* **2017**, *19*(4), 2573-
       2620.
       [http://dx.doi.org/10.1109/COMST.2017.2731979]

[59]   Choi, Y.; Parsani, R.; Pandey, A.V.; Roman, X.; Cheok, A.D. *Light Perfume* : A Fashion Accessory
       for Synchronization of Nonverbal Communication. *Leonardo,* **2013**, *46*(5), 439-444.

[http://dx.doi.org/10.1162/LEON_a_00638]

[60]   Abbasi, J. Skin-like Wearable Health Monitors. *JAMA,* **2017**, *318*(14), 1314.
       [http://dx.doi.org/10.1001/jama.2017.14440] [PMID: 29049568]

[61]   Gentleman, R.C.; Carey, V.J.; Bates, D.M.; Bolstad, B.; Dettling, M.; Dudoit, S.; Ellis, B.; Gautier, L.;
       Ge, Y.; Gentry, J.; Hornik, K.; Hothorn, T.; Huber, W.; Iacus, S.; Irizarry, R.; Leisch, F.; Li, C.;
       Maechler, M.; Rossini, A.J.; Sawitzki, G.; Smith, C.; Smyth, G.; Tierney, L.; Yang, J.Y.H.; Zhang, J.
       Bioconductor: open software development for computational biology and bioinformatics. *Genome
       Biol.,* **2004**, *5*(10), R80.
       [http://dx.doi.org/10.1186/gb-2004-5-10-r80] [PMID: 15461798]

[62]   Dunn, B.; Kamath, H.; Tarascon, J.M. Electrical energy storage for the grid: a battery of choices.
       Science, **2011**, *334*(6058), 928-935.
       [http://dx.doi.org/10.1126/science.1212741] [PMID: 22096188]

[63]   Bakker, C.; Wang, F.; Huisman, J.; den Hollander, M. Products that go round: exploring product life
       extension through design. *J. Clean. Prod.,* **2014**, *69*, 10-16.
       [http://dx.doi.org/10.1016/j.jclepro.2014.01.028]

[64]   Goldstein, C.A.; Berry, R.B.; Kent, D.T.; Kristo, D.A.; Seixas, A.A.; Redline, S.; Westover, M.B.
       Artificial intelligence in sleep medicine: background and implications for clinicians. *J. Clin. Sleep
       Med.,* **2020**, *16*(4), 609-618.
       [http://dx.doi.org/10.5664/jcsm.8388] [PMID: 32065113]

[65]   Seneviratne, S.; Hu, Y.; Nguyen, T.; Lan, G.; Khalifa, S.; Thilakarathna, K.; Hassan, M.; Seneviratne,
       A. A Survey of Wearable Devices and Challenges. *IEEE Commun. Surv. Tutor.,* **2017**, *19*(4), 2573-
       2620.
       [http://dx.doi.org/10.1109/COMST.2017.2731979]

CHAPTER 4

Nanotechnology in Construction and Infrastructure

Abstract: Nanotechnology is rapidly transforming the construction and infrastructure sectors by introducing advanced materials and innovative techniques that enhance performance, sustainability, and safety. This chapter explores the critical applications of nanotechnology in construction, focusing on stronger and lighter materials, self-healing concrete, and sustainable practices. The use of nanomaterials, such as carbon nanotubes and nano-silica, improves the strength, durability, and efficiency of construction materials, while lightweight nanocomposites offer structural advantages. Self-healing concrete, enabled by nanotechnology, reduces maintenance costs and extends the lifespan of infrastructure. Additionally, nanotechnology's role in sustainable construction practices, including thermal insulation, water purification, and environmental protection, is highlighted. The role of nanotechnology in smart cities and future trends in civil engineering are also discussed. Safety considerations and regulatory frameworks are crucial to ensuring the responsible use of nanomaterials in construction. Real-world case studies demonstrate the impact of nanotechnology on construction efficiency, sustainability, and overall project success. This chapter provides a comprehensive overview of how nanotechnology is reshaping the construction industry and paving the way for more resilient and eco-friendly infrastructure.

Keywords: Construction, Infrastructure, Lightweight, Material science, Nanocomposites, Nanomaterials.

INTRODUCTION

Nanotechnology has rapidly emerged as a transformative force in the construction industry, offering innovative solutions that enhance the performance, durability, and sustainability of construction materials and infrastructure, as listed in Table **4.1**. These properties include enhanced strength, lighter weight, improved resistance to environmental degradation, and increased energy efficiency [1]. In construction, nanotechnology is applied in various areas, such as the development of nanomaterials like nano-concrete, nanocomposites, and nano-coatings. Nano-concrete, for instance, utilizes nanoparticles to enhance the mechanical properties of concrete, making it stronger, more durable, and less prone to cracking. Nanocomposites, which combine nanomaterials with traditional construction

Shivang Dhoundiyal & Aftab Alam

materials, offer improved load-bearing capabilities while reducing the overall weight of structures. Nano-coatings are used to protect surfaces from wear, corrosion, and even microbial growth, extending the lifespan of buildings and infrastructure [2]. Nanotechnology also plays a pivotal role in the development of smart materials and systems, such as self-cleaning surfaces and energy-efficient insulation. These innovations contribute to more sustainable construction practices by reducing energy consumption, minimizing waste, and lowering maintenance costs. The use of nanotechnology in construction is not limited to materials alone; it extends to advanced sensors and monitoring systems that enable real-time tracking of structural health, thereby enhancing safety and reducing the risk of catastrophic failures [3]. The importance of nanotechnology in modern infrastructure cannot be overstated, as it addresses many of the critical challenges faced by the construction industry today. One of the primary benefits of nanotechnology is its ability to enhance the mechanical properties of construction materials. By improving the strength-to-weight ratio of materials, nanotechnology allows for the creation of structures that are both lighter and stronger, enabling the construction of taller buildings, longer bridges, and more expansive infrastructure projects without compromising safety or stability. In addition to improving material performance, nanotechnology contributes to the sustainability of modern infrastructure. The construction industry is a significant contributor to global carbon emissions, and nanotechnology offers solutions to reduce the environmental impact of construction activities. For example, the development of nano-cement with lower carbon footprints, self-healing materials that reduce the need for frequent repairs, and energy-efficient insulation materials that reduce energy consumption in buildings are all examples of how nanotechnology can support the construction of greener, more sustainable infrastructure [4]. Nanotechnology also plays a crucial role in enhancing the longevity and durability of infrastructure. Traditional construction materials are susceptible to degradation over time due to factors such as weathering, corrosion, and chemical exposure. Nanomaterials, with their enhanced resistance to these factors, can extend the lifespan of infrastructure, reducing the need for costly repairs and replacements. This not only lowers the overall cost of infrastructure maintenance but also ensures the safety and reliability of critical structures. Nanotechnology enables the development of smart infrastructure that can adapt to changing conditions and provide real-time data on structural health [5]. For instance, nanosensors embedded in concrete can monitor stress, temperature, and other factors that affect the integrity of a structure, allowing for timely interventions before failures occur. This capability is particularly important in areas prone to natural disasters, where early detection of structural issues can save lives and prevent catastrophic damage.

Table 4.1. Applications of nanotechnology in construction and infrastructure.

Application Area	Nanotechnology Innovation	Benefits	Examples/Case Studies	References
Stronger and Lighter Materials	Nanomaterials like carbon nanotubes, nano-silica, and graphene.	Enhanced strength, reduced weight, and improved durability.	Donghai Bridge (China) using nano-silica in concrete.	[6]
Self-healing Concrete	Nano-encapsulated healing agents, bacteria-based nanomaterials.	Automatic crack repair, extended lifespan, and reduced maintenance costs.	University of Cambridge's self-healing concrete research.	[7]
Sustainable Construction Practices	Nanomaterials for energy efficiency and green building materials.	Reduced carbon footprint and better resource utilization.	Masdar City (UAE) uses nano-insulation for energy-efficient buildings.	[8]
Thermal Insulation and Energy Efficiency	Aerogels and nano-porous materials.	Superior thermal insulation and reduced energy consumption.	Aerogel insulation in commercial and residential buildings.	[9]
Water Purification and Environmental Protection	Nano-filtration systems, photocatalytic coatings.	Clean water, pollution control, and improved environmental impact.	Photocatalytic TiO_2 coatings for air purification on building facades.	[10]
Smart Infrastructure	Embedded nano-sensors, nano-coatings for durability	Real-time monitoring, adaptive infrastructure.	Smart cities like Masdar are integrating nanosensors for environmental monitoring.	[11]

STRONGER AND LIGHTER MATERIALS

Nanomaterials are at the forefront of advancements in construction, offering unparalleled improvements in strength and durability. These materials are engineered at the nanoscale, where they exhibit unique properties that traditional construction materials cannot match. For instance, the addition of carbon nanotubes (CNTs) or graphene to concrete and steel significantly enhances their mechanical properties [12]. CNTs, known for their extraordinary tensile strength, are incorporated into cement to create nano-concrete that is not only stronger but also more resistant to cracking and deformation. This enhanced strength reduces the need for large amounts of raw materials, leading to more efficient construction processes. Moreover, nanomaterials contribute to the durability of construction materials by making them more resistant to environmental factors such as moisture, temperature fluctuations, and chemical exposure. For example, nano-silica particles added to concrete reduce its porosity, making it less susceptible to water infiltration and the subsequent freeze-thaw cycles that can cause cracking [13]. Additionally, nano-coatings applied to steel structures can protect them from corrosion, significantly extending their lifespan in harsh environments. The ability of nanomaterials to enhance both strength and durability is critical for constructing long-lasting infrastructure that requires minimal maintenance over time. Lightweight nanocomposites are revolutionizing the construction industry by enabling the creation of structures that are both strong and light [14]. Traditional construction materials, such as concrete and steel, often add significant weight to buildings and infrastructure, limiting design possibilities and requiring substantial foundational support. However, nanocomposites, which combine nanoparticles with conventional materials, offer a solution by providing the same or even greater strength while drastically reducing weight. For example, carbon nanofibers or nanoparticles can be integrated into polymer matrices to create nanocomposites with exceptional mechanical properties. These materials are not only lightweight but also exhibit high stiffness, making them ideal for load-bearing applications. In the construction of bridges, skyscrapers, and other large-scale infrastructure projects, lightweight nanocomposites allow for more innovative and flexible designs while reducing the overall load on the structure. This weight reduction also translates to lower transportation and installation costs, further enhancing the efficiency of construction projects [15]. Additionally, lightweight nanocomposites are particularly valuable in seismic zones, where the reduced weight of structures can minimize the impact of earthquakes. By incorporating these advanced materials, engineers can design buildings and infrastructure that are both resilient and capable of withstanding extreme conditions without sacrificing strength. The practical application of stronger and lighter nanomaterials in construction is already underway, with numerous case studies demonstrating their effectiveness. One notable example is the use of nano-silica in the construction of the Willis Tower (formerly known as the Sears Tower) in Chicago [16]. By incorporating nano-silica into the concrete mix, engineers were able to reduce the building's overall weight while increasing the strength of the concrete. This allowed for a more efficient design that supported the tower's height and withstood the stresses of wind and seismic activity. Another example is the use of carbon nanotubes in the construction of bridges. In Japan, CNT-reinforced concrete has been used in the construction of several bridges, including the Akashi Kaikyō Bridge, one of the longest suspension bridges in the world [17]. The integration of CNTs provided the concrete with enhanced tensile strength and durability, ensuring that the bridge can withstand the harsh marine environment and the dynamic loads imposed by traffic and wind. In addition to these large-scale projects, nanomaterials have also been successfully implemented in smaller, specialized applications. For instance, nano-coatings have been applied to steel structures in offshore oil rigs, where corrosion is a significant concern. These nano-coatings provide a protective barrier that prevents rust and extends the lifespan of the structures, reducing maintenance costs and minimizing environmental impact [18]. These case studies highlight the transformative potential of nanomaterials in construction, demonstrating how they can lead to stronger, lighter, and more durable structures.

SELF-HEALING CONCRETE

Self-healing concrete is an innovative material designed to automatically repair cracks and damage without the need for human intervention. This concept is inspired by biological systems, where self-repair mechanisms are common, such as the healing of a broken bone. In construction, cracks in concrete are a major issue as they allow water, chemicals, and other harmful agents to penetrate the structure, leading to further deterioration over time. Self-healing concrete addresses this problem by integrating mechanisms that activate upon the appearance of cracks, effectively "healing" the damage and restoring the material's integrity [19]. The mechanism of self-healing concrete can vary, but one of the most common approaches involves the use of encapsulated healing agents. Microcapsules containing materials such as liquid healing agents (*e.g.,* epoxy, polyurethane) or bacteria are embedded within the concrete matrix during the mixing process [20]. When a crack forms, these microcapsules rupture, releasing their contents into the crack. The healing agent then solidifies, filling the crack and preventing further damage. In the case of bacteria-based self-healing concrete, the bacteria are activated by water entering the crack, triggering a chemical reaction that produces calcium carbonate, which fills and seals the crack. Another approach involves the use of shape-memory materials or polymers that respond to external stimuli, such as temperature changes, to close cracks [21]. These materials can expand or contract to fill gaps in the concrete when triggered, effectively repairing the damage. The concept of self-healing concrete represents a significant advancement in materials science, offering a way to extend the lifespan of structures and reduce maintenance costs.

Nanomaterials play a crucial role in enhancing the effectiveness of self-healing concrete. These materials, due to their small size and large surface area, can interact with the concrete matrix at a molecular level, improving the material's self-healing capabilities. One of the most widely used nanomaterials in self-healing concrete is nano-silica. Nano-silica particles can improve the density and strength of the concrete, making it more resistant to cracking. Additionally, when cracks occur, nano-silica can help fill the voids and promote the formation of calcium silicate hydrate (C-S-H), a key component in the healing process [22].

Another important nanomaterial used in self-healing concrete is titanium dioxide (TiO_2). TiO_2 nanoparticles not only enhance the mechanical properties of concrete but also have photocatalytic properties, which can help in the degradation of pollutants that may enter cracks. This makes the concrete self-healing and self-cleaning, adding another layer of functionality to the material. Carbon-based nanomaterials, such as carbon nanotubes (CNTs) and graphene, are also used to improve the self-healing properties of concrete. CNTs can reinforce the concrete matrix, making it more resilient to cracking, while graphene can enhance the conductivity of the concrete, allowing for the use of electrical or thermal stimuli to activate healing mechanisms. Bacterial spores encapsulated in nanoscale materials are another innovative approach [23]. These spores remain dormant until activated by moisture from cracks, at which point they produce limestone to seal the cracks. The use of nanomaterials in self-healing concrete enhances its performance, making it a more viable solution for long-lasting infrastructure. The advantages of self-healing concrete are numerous and impactful, particularly in the context of infrastructure sustainability and cost reduction. One of the primary benefits is the significant extension of the lifespan of concrete structures. Traditional concrete is prone to cracking over time due to environmental factors such as temperature fluctuations, moisture, and load stress. Self-healing concrete mitigates these issues by automatically repairing small cracks before they can grow into larger problems, reducing the need for costly repairs and maintenance [24]. This can result in substantial cost savings over the lifetime of a structure. Another advantage is the enhanced durability and resilience of structures made with self-healing concrete. By maintaining structural integrity over time, self-healing concrete contributes to the safety of buildings, bridges, roads, and other critical infrastructure. In addition, self-healing concrete offers environmental benefits by reducing the need for raw materials and energy-intensive repair processes [25]. This aligns with the goals of sustainable construction, where minimizing waste and lowering carbon footprints are key objectives. However, the implementation of self-healing concrete is not without challenges. One of the main challenges is the cost associated with the initial production of self-healing materials. The function of microcapsules, bacteria, or nanomaterials in concrete can increase the overall cost, which may be a barrier for widespread adoption, especially in budget-constrained projects. Additionally, there are concerns about the long-term performance and reliability of self-healing mechanisms, particularly in harsh environments. While laboratory tests have shown promising results, real-world conditions can be more variable, and there is still ongoing research to ensure that self-healing concrete performs consistently over time. The scalability of self-healing concrete production is another challenge. Developing methods to produce self-healing concrete on a large scale, while maintaining cost-effectiveness and quality, is a complex task that requires further innovation and investment [26]. Addressing these challenges will be crucial for the broader adoption of self-healing concrete in the construction industry. Several real-world applications have demonstrated the potential of self-healing concrete in various infrastructure projects. One notable example is the application of self-healing concrete in the construction of the Dutch motorway, the A58. In this project, self-healing concrete was used in the pavement to prevent the formation of cracks and potholes, which are common issues in road construction [27]. The self-healing properties of the concrete allowed for the automatic repair of minor cracks caused by traffic loads and weather conditions, reducing the need for frequent maintenance and increasing the road's lifespan. Another case study involves the use of bacterial self-healing concrete in the construction of water-retaining structures in the Netherlands. In these structures, self-healing concrete was employed to address the issue of water leakage through cracks. The bacteria in the concrete were activated by moisture, leading to the production of calcium carbonate that sealed the cracks and prevented water from penetrating the structure. This application was particularly beneficial in a water-rich environment, where the durability and integrity of the structures were critical for preventing leaks and maintaining water quality. In the United Kingdom, self-healing concrete has been tested in bridge construction as part of the Materials for Life (M4L) project [28]. This research initiative explored various self-healing technologies, including encapsulated healing agents and shape-memory materials, to improve the longevity and resilience of bridges. The project demonstrated that self-healing concrete could significantly reduce the occurrence of cracks and extend the service life of bridges, contributing to more sustainable infrastructure. These case studies highlight the practical benefits of self-healing concrete in real-world applications, showing how it can improve the durability, safety, and sustainability of construction projects.

INNOVATIONS IN CIVIL ENGINEERING

Nanotechnology is increasingly becoming a key driver in the movement toward sustainable construction practices. The construction industry is known for its significant environmental impact, contributing to large amounts of waste, energy consumption, and greenhouse gas emissions. Nanotechnology offers innovative solutions to mitigate these impacts by enhancing material efficiency, reducing resource consumption, and improving the environmental performance of buildings and infrastructure. One of the primary ways nanotechnology contributes to sustainability in construction is through the development of materials that require fewer raw resources and offer longer lifespans [29]. For instance, nanomaterials can strengthen concrete and steel, allowing for thinner and lighter structures that maintain or even exceed the performance of traditional materials. This reduction in material use not only conserves resources but also decreases transportation and construction costs, leading to more efficient building practices. Nanotechnology enables the creation of smart and adaptive materials that respond to environmental conditions. For example, self-cleaning and self-healing materials reduce the need for maintenance and repairs, thereby lowering the overall lifecycle cost and environmental footprint of buildings. Nano-coatings can also improve the durability of materials by making them resistant to corrosion, UV radiation, and other forms of degradation, further contributing to sustainability [30]. Nanotechnology also plays a crucial role in the development of energy-efficient buildings. By improving insulation, energy storage, and energy generation, nanotechnology supports the construction of green buildings that consume less energy and reduce carbon emissions. Nanomaterials are revolutionizing the field of thermal insulation and energy efficiency in construction. Buildings account for a large percentage of global energy consumption, particularly in heating and cooling. Traditional insulation materials, while effective, have limitations in terms of thickness, weight, and performance. Nanomaterials, with their unique properties, offer enhanced insulation capabilities, leading to more energy-efficient buildings. One of the most promising nanomaterials for insulation is aerogel, often referred to as "frozen smoke" due to its lightweight and porous structure [31]. Aerogels have extremely low thermal conductivity, making them excellent insulators. Despite being lightweight and thin, aerogels provide superior insulation compared to traditional materials like fiberglass or foam. This makes them ideal for applications where space and weight are critical factors, such as in retrofitting older buildings or in modern construction where thin walls are desired. Another important nanomaterial for insulation is nano-porous silica. Like aerogel, it has a high surface area and low thermal conductivity, allowing it to trap air and prevent heat transfer. Nano-porous silica can be incorporated into panels or coatings, providing efficient thermal insulation while maintaining a lightweight profile [32]. This material is particularly useful in improving the energy efficiency of walls, roofs, and windows. In addition to improving insulation, nanomaterials also contribute to energy efficiency by enhancing the performance of energy-generating systems. For example, nanotechnology is used to create thin, flexible solar panels that can be integrated into building facades or rooftops. These panels capture solar energy and convert it into electricity, reducing the building's reliance on external power sources and lowering energy bills. Nanotechnology is playing a critical role in advancing water purification and environmental protection efforts, particularly within the construction industry. Water is a vital resource, and ensuring its purity and availability is essential for both human health and the environment. Construction activities often contribute to water pollution through runoff, chemical leaching, and waste [33]. Nanotechnology offers innovative solutions to address these challenges by providing advanced water purification systems and materials that minimize environmental impact.

Nanomaterials, such as carbon nanotubes and graphene, have been developed for use in water filtration and purification systems. These materials have exceptional adsorption capacities, allowing them to remove contaminants such as heavy metals, bacteria, and organic pollutants from water. For instance, carbon nanotubes can filter out pollutants at the molecular level, making them highly effective in producing clean water [34]. These nanomaterials can be integrated into filtration membranes used in construction projects, ensuring that water used on-site is purified and free from harmful substances. Another application of nanotechnology in water purification is the development of photocatalytic materials, such as titanium dioxide (TiO_2) nanoparticles. When exposed to sunlight, TiO_2 nanoparticles generate reactive oxygen species that break down organic pollutants and kill bacteria in water [35]. This photocatalytic process can be used to treat wastewater generated during construction activities, preventing contaminants from entering natural water sources and protecting aquatic ecosystems. In addition to water purification, nanotechnology contributes to environmental protection by providing materials that minimize pollution and waste. For example, nano-coatings applied to construction materials can prevent the release of harmful chemicals into the environment. These coatings can also make surfaces self-cleaning, reducing the need for chemical cleaning agents that could pollute water sources.

Smart Infrastructure and Future Perspectives

The concept of smart infrastructure is central to the development of smart cities, where technology is seamlessly integrated into urban systems to improve efficiency, sustainability, and the quality of life for residents. Nanotechnology plays a pivotal role in enabling smart infrastructure by providing advanced materials and systems that enhance the functionality and resilience of urban environments. In smart cities, nanotechnology is used to create intelligent buildings, responsive transportation networks, and sustainable energy systems that are all interconnected through the Internet of Things (IoT) [36]. One of the key applications of nanotechnology in smart infrastructure is in the development of smart materials that can sense and respond to environmental changes. For instance, nanomaterials can be embedded in concrete to monitor structural health in real-time. These materials can detect stress, strain, and even microscopic cracks, allowing for early intervention before significant damage occurs. This proactive approach to infrastructure maintenance not only enhances safety but also reduces the cost of repairs and extends the lifespan of buildings, bridges, and roads. Nanotechnology also contributes to the energy efficiency of smart cities. Nano-enhanced solar panels, for example, can be integrated into building facades, windows, and even roads to generate clean energy. Additionally, nanomaterials are used in energy storage systems, such as advanced batteries and supercapacitors, to provide efficient power management for smart grids. These innovations ensure that smart cities can meet their energy needs sustainably, reducing their reliance on fossil fuels and minimizing their carbon footprint. In transportation, nanotechnology is used to develop lightweight, strong, and durable materials for vehicles and infrastructure [37]. This leads to more efficient public transit systems, reduced energy consumption, and lower emissions. Smart sensors powered by nanotechnology are also employed in traffic management systems to optimize traffic flow, reduce congestion, and improve road safety.

The future of civil engineering is poised to be transformed by the continued advancement of nanotechnology. One of the most promising trends in nanotechnology for civil engineering is the development of multifunctional materials. These materials, which combine several properties into a single system, are expected to play a significant role in the future of construction, as illustrated in Fig (**4.1**). For example, researchers are exploring nanomaterials that not only provide structural support but also offer self-healing, energy-harvesting, and pollution-removing capabilities [38]. These multifunctional materials could lead to buildings and infrastructure that are more sustainable, self-sufficient, and capable of adapting to environmental changes. Another emerging trend is the use of nanotechnology to enhance the resilience of infrastructure against natural disasters. Nanomaterials are being developed to improve the strength and flexibility of structures, making them more resistant to earthquakes, floods, and extreme weather events. For instance, nanocomposites can be used to reinforce concrete and steel, enabling buildings and bridges to withstand greater forces without compromising safety. Additionally, nanotechnology is being explored for use in disaster detection and early warning systems, with nanosensors that can monitor environmental conditions and provide real-time data on potential hazards. The convergence of nanotechnology with other cutting-edge technologies, such as artificial intelligence (AI) and robotics, is also expected to shape the future of civil engineering. For example, AI-driven algorithms can analyze data from nanomaterial sensors embedded in infrastructure to predict maintenance needs and optimize construction processes [39]. Robotics, powered by nanotechnology, can be used for precision construction and repairs, reducing human labor and increasing efficiency. Sustainability will continue to be a driving force behind the future of nanotechnology in civil engineering. As the construction industry faces increasing pressure to reduce its environmental impact, nanotechnology will be crucial in developing eco-friendly materials and processes. For example, researchers are working on nanomaterials that can capture and store carbon dioxide, reducing greenhouse gas emissions from construction activities [40]. Additionally, innovations in water purification, waste management, and energy efficiency, driven by nanotechnology, will contribute to more sustainable infrastructure.

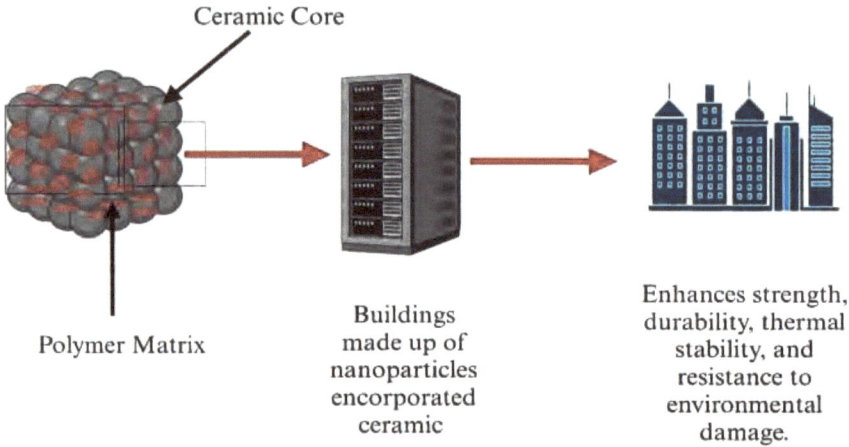

Fig. (4.1). Nanoparticles incorporated into ceramics can help reduce damage and strain.

REAL-WORLD APPLICATIONS

Nanotechnology has already made its mark on several high-profile infrastructure projects around the world, showcasing its potential to revolutionize the construction industry. These real-world applications provide concrete examples of how nanomaterials and nanotechnology innovations are being used to create stronger, more durable, and sustainable infrastructure. One notable example is the use of nano-engineered concrete in the construction of bridges and highways. For instance, the Donghai Bridge in China, one of the longest cross-sea bridges in the world, incorporates nanomaterials to enhance the strength and durability of the concrete [41]. By adding nano-silica particles, the concrete used in the bridge has higher resistance to cracking, improved compressive strength, and better longevity in harsh marine environments. This application demonstrates how nanotechnology can extend the lifespan of critical infrastructure while reducing maintenance costs. Another example is the application of self-cleaning nano-coatings on the exterior of buildings. The Torre Agbar skyscraper in Barcelona, Spain, utilizes a titanium dioxide (TiO_2) nano-coating on its façade [42]. This coating reacts with sunlight to break down pollutants and organic matter, keeping the building clean without the need for regular washing. The self-cleaning properties of the coating not only reduce maintenance costs but also contribute to environmental sustainability by minimizing the use of water and cleaning chemicals. Nanotechnology is also being applied in smart infrastructure projects. The city of Masdar in the United Arab Emirates, designed to be a sustainable, zero-carbon city, integrates nanomaterials in various aspects of its construction [43]. For example, nano-insulation materials are used to improve the energy efficiency of buildings, while nano-sensors monitor environmental conditions and energy usage in real-time.

These applications illustrate how nanotechnology can be harnessed to create smart, sustainable urban environments. In addition to these large-scale projects, nanotechnology is making its way into everyday infrastructure improvements. For example, nano-enabled asphalt is being used in road construction to create more durable and weather-resistant surfaces. In cities like Los Angeles, roads treated with nano-additives have shown increased resistance to cracking and wear, leading to longer-lasting roads that require less frequent repairs [44]. These case studies highlight the growing impact of nanotechnology on infrastructure projects worldwide. From bridges and skyscrapers to roads and smart cities, nanotechnology is enabling the construction of more advanced, resilient, and sustainable infrastructure. Nanotechnology has a profound impact on construction efficiency and sustainability, transforming traditional building practices and materials, as depicted in Fig. **(4.2)**. By incorporating nanomaterials into construction processes, the industry can achieve greater efficiency, reduce waste, and minimize the environmental footprint of infrastructure projects. One of the most significant impacts of nanotechnology on construction efficiency is the development of stronger and lighter materials [45]. Nanomaterials, such as carbon nanotubes and nano-silica, are used to enhance the properties of concrete, steel, and other building materials. These enhanced materials require less raw material to achieve the same or better performance compared to traditional materials. This reduction in material usage not only conserves natural resources but also leads to cost savings in transportation, handling, and installation. For example, nano-enhanced concrete can achieve the same strength with less cement, reducing the amount of energy-intensive cement production and lowering carbon emissions [46]. Nanotechnology also improves construction efficiency through the creation of self-healing materials. Self-healing concrete, for instance, can automatically repair cracks and damage, reducing the need for frequent maintenance and repairs. This innovation extends the lifespan of infrastructure, decreases downtime, and minimizes the labour and resources required for upkeep. By reducing maintenance demands, nanotechnology contributes to more efficient and cost-effective construction practices [47]. In terms of sustainability, nanotechnology enables the construction of eco-friendly buildings and infrastructure. Nano-insulation materials, such as aerogels and nano-porous silica, offer superior thermal performance, reducing the energy consumption required for heating and cooling. These materials contribute to the development of energy-efficient buildings that lower carbon emissions and reduce reliance on fossil fuels. Additionally, nano-coatings and surface treatments can make materials more resistant to environmental degradation, extending their lifespan and reducing the need for replacements. Nanotechnology also supports sustainable water and waste management practices in construction. Nano-filtration systems can purify water used on construction sites, ensuring that contaminants do not pollute nearby water sources. Nano-enabled sensors can monitor water usage, helping construction managers optimize water consumption and reduce waste [48]. These technologies contribute to more responsible resource management and minimize the environmental impact of construction activities. Nanotechnology enhances construction sustainability by enabling the development of green building materials. For example, researchers are exploring the use of nanocellulose, a biodegradable material derived from plant fibers, as a sustainable alternative to traditional construction materials. Nanocellulose has excellent mechanical properties and can be used in a variety of applications, from lightweight composites to eco-friendly insulation.

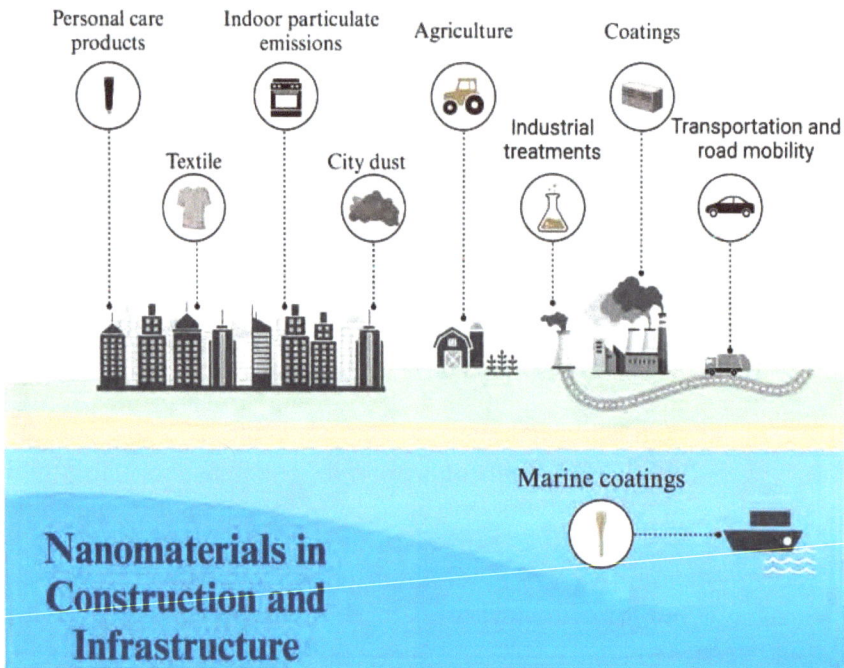

Fig. (4.2). Various domains where nanoparticles play a significant role.

SAFETY AND REGULATORY ASPECTS

The use of nanomaterials in construction brings forth several safety considerations that need to be addressed to protect workers, end-users, and the environment. As nanomaterials are engineered at an atomic or molecular scale, they can exhibit unique properties, such as increased reactivity or biological interactions, that may pose potential risks if not properly managed. One of the primary safety concerns associated with nanomaterials is their potential impact on human health. Workers handling nanomaterials during construction activities may be exposed to nanoparticles through inhalation, skin contact, or ingestion [49]. Due to their small size, nanoparticles can penetrate deep into the respiratory system, potentially causing respiratory issues, inflammation, or even more severe health problems. Additionally, some nanomaterials may exhibit cytotoxicity, leading to adverse effects on cellular functions. To mitigate these risks, it is essential to implement strict safety protocols, including the use of personal protective equipment (PPE) such as masks, gloves, and protective clothing, as well as proper ventilation systems to minimize exposure. Another safety consideration is the environmental impact of nanomaterials. During construction, nanomaterials may be released into the environment through dust, waste, or runoff, potentially contaminating soil, water, and air. The persistence and bioaccumulation of certain nanomaterials in ecosystems can lead to long-term environmental effects. For instance, nanoparticles in water systems may be ingested by aquatic organisms, leading to toxic effects and disruption of the food chain [50]. To address these concerns, proper waste management practices must be implemented, including the containment and disposal of nanomaterial waste per environmental regulations. The long-term safety of nanomaterials in construction is another area of concern. As many nanomaterials are relatively new, their long-term behavior and potential degradation over time are not yet fully understood. For example, the breakdown of nanomaterials in building materials could lead to the release of nanoparticles into indoor environments, potentially impacting the health of occupants. Therefore, ongoing research and monitoring are needed to assess the long-term safety of nanomaterials and to develop guidelines for their safe use in construction projects. In conclusion, while nanomaterials offer significant benefits for construction, their safety considerations must be carefully managed. Ensuring the health and safety of workers, protecting the environment, and understanding the long-term effects of nanomaterials are critical steps in the responsible use of nanotechnology in the construction industry [51]. At the international level, several organizations are working to establish standards for nanomaterials in construction. The International Organization for Standardization (ISO) and the International Electrotechnical Commission (IEC) have developed standards related to the terminology, characterization, and safety of nanomaterials [52]. These standards provide a common framework for the classification and measurement of nanomaterials, helping to ensure consistency and transparency in their use across different industries, including construction. In addition to international standards, national regulatory agencies are also establishing guidelines for the use of nanomaterials in infrastructure projects. For example, the European Union has implemented regulations that require manufacturers and suppliers of nanomaterials to provide detailed information on their properties, potential hazards, and safe handling practices. The EU's Registration, Evaluation, Authorization, and Restriction of Chemicals (REACH) regulation specifically addresses nanomaterials, requiring that they be registered and assessed for safety before being placed on the market [53]. This ensures that nanomaterials used in construction are thoroughly evaluated for their potential risks to human health and the environment. In the United States, the Environmental Protection Agency (EPA) and the Occupational Safety and Health Administration (OSHA) have established guidelines for the safe use of nanomaterials in various industries, including construction. The EPA has developed regulations for the testing and evaluation of nanomaterials under the Toxic Substances Control Act (TSCA), while OSHA guides workplace safety measures to protect workers from exposure to nanoparticles [54]. These regulations help ensure that nanomaterials are used safely and responsibly in construction projects. Despite the progress made in developing regulatory frameworks for nanotechnology in construction, challenges remain. The rapid pace of innovation in nanotechnology often outstrips the ability of regulatory agencies to keep up with new developments. Additionally, the diverse range of nanomaterials and their applications in construction requires a flexible and adaptive regulatory approach [55]. Ongoing collaboration between industry, academia, and regulatory bodies is essential to address these challenges and to ensure that regulations remain relevant and effective.

CONCLUSION

Nanotechnology is poised to revolutionize the construction industry by offering innovative solutions that address both traditional and emerging challenges. Stronger and lighter nanomaterials, such as carbon nanotubes and nano-silica, are enabling the creation of more durable and efficient infrastructure, while self-healing concrete is minimizing the need for repairs and extending the lifespan of buildings and roads. Nanotechnology is also driving sustainable construction practices by improving energy efficiency, water purification, and environmental protection. As smart cities become more prevalent, the integration of nanotechnology will be essential for developing intelligent and adaptive infrastructure. However, the widespread adoption of nanotechnology in construction requires careful attention to safety and regulatory standards to mitigate potential risks. Through real-world applications, it is evident that nanotechnology is enhancing construction efficiency and sustainability, making it a critical component of modern infrastructure development. As the industry continues to evolve, the future of construction will undoubtedly be shaped by the ongoing advancements in nanotechnology.

REFERENCES

[1]   Tamaki, R.; Tanaka, Y.; Asuncion, M.Z.; Choi, J.; Laine, R.M. Octa(aminophenyl)silsesquioxane as a Nanoconstruction Site. *J. Am. Chem. Soc.,* **2001,** *123*(49), 12416-12417.
        [http://dx.doi.org/10.1021/ja011781m] [PMID: 11734046]

[2] Besinis, A.; De Peralta, T.; Handy, R.D. Inhibition of biofilm formation and antibacterial properties of a silver nano-coating on human dentine. *Nanotoxicology,* **2013**, 1-10.
[http://dx.doi.org/10.3109/17435390.2013.825343] [PMID: 23875717]

[3] Hasan, S. abdalkhaliq. The Use of Nanotechnology in Construction Sector. *Al-Qadisiyah Journal for Engineering Sciences,* **2014**, *7*(1), 68-80.

[4] Aricò, A.S.; Bruce, P.; Scrosati, B.; Tarascon, J.M.; van Schalkwijk, W. Nanostructured materials for advanced energy conversion and storage devices. *Nat. Mater.,* **2005**, *4*(5), 366-377.
[http://dx.doi.org/10.1038/nmat1368] [PMID: 15867920]

[5] Klaine, S.J.; Koelmans, A.A.; Horne, N.; Carley, S.; Handy, R.D.; Kapustka, L.; Nowack, B.; von der Kammer, F. Paradigms to assess the environmental impact of manufactured nanomaterials. *Environ. Toxicol. Chem.,* **2012**, *31*(1), 3-14.
[http://dx.doi.org/10.1002/etc.733] [PMID: 22162122]

[6] Moskvitina, E.; Kuznetsov, V.; Moseenkov, S.; Serkova, A.; Zavorin, A. Antibacterial Effect of Carbon Nanomaterials: Nanotubes, Carbon Nanofibers, Nanodiamonds, and Onion-like Carbon. *Materials (Basel),* **2023**, *16*(3), 957-957.
[http://dx.doi.org/10.3390/ma16030957] [PMID: 36769964]

[7] Wang, J.Y.; Soens, H.; Verstraete, W.; De Belie, N. Self-healing concrete by use of microencapsulated bacterial spores. *Cement Concr. Res.,* **2014**, *56*, 139-152.
[http://dx.doi.org/10.1016/j.cemconres.2013.11.009]

[8] Serrano, E.; Rus, G.; García-Martínez, J. Nanotechnology for sustainable energy. *Renew. Sustain. Energy Rev.,* **2009**, *13*(9), 2373-2384.
[http://dx.doi.org/10.1016/j.rser.2009.06.003]

[9] Prediction of the Effective Thermal Conductivity of Aerogel Nano-Porous Materials *Energy Procedia,* **2017**, *105*, 4769-4775.
[http://dx.doi.org/10.1016/j.egypro.2017.03.938]

[10] Sharma, V.K.; Yngard, R.A.; Lin, Y. Silver nanoparticles: Green synthesis and their antimicrobial activities. *Adv. Colloid Interface Sci.,* **2009**, *145*(1-2), 83-96.
[http://dx.doi.org/10.1016/j.cis.2008.09.002] [PMID: 18945421]

[11] Ye, S.; Rathmell, A.R.; Chen, Z.; Stewart, I.E.; Wiley, B.J. Metal nanowire networks: the next generation of transparent conductors. *Adv. Mater.,* **2014**, *26*(39), 6670-6687.
[http://dx.doi.org/10.1002/adma.201402710] [PMID: 25252266]

[12] Golberg, D.; Bando, Y.; Huang, Y.; Terao, T.; Mitome, M.; Tang, C.; Zhi, C. Boron nitride nanotubes and nanosheets. *ACS Nano,* **2010**, *4*(6), 2979-2993.
[http://dx.doi.org/10.1021/nn1006495] [PMID: 20462272]

[13] Zhang, P.; Sha, D.; Li, Q.; Zhao, S.; Ling, Y. Effect of nano silica particles on impact resistance and durability of concrete containing coal fly ash. *Nanomaterials (Basel),* **2021**, *11*(5), 1296.
[http://dx.doi.org/10.3390/nano11051296] [PMID: 34069094]

[14] Thomas, B.; Raj, M.C.; B, A.K.; H, R.M.; Joy, J.; Moores, A.; Drisko, G.L.; Sanchez, C. Nanocellulose, a Versatile Green Platform: From Biosources to Materials and Their Applications. *Chem. Rev.,* **2018**, *118*(24), 11575-11625.
[http://dx.doi.org/10.1021/acs.chemrev.7b00627] [PMID: 30403346]

[15] D'Alessandro, D.M.; Smit, B.; Long, J.R. Carbon Dioxide Capture: Prospects for New Materials. *Angew. Chem. Int. Ed.,* **2010**, *49*(35), 6058-6082.
[http://dx.doi.org/10.1002/anie.201000431]

[16] Oliver, W.C.; Pharr, G.M. An improved technique for determining hardness and elastic modulus using load and displacement sensing indentation experiments. *J. Mater. Res.,* **1992**, *7*(6), 1564-1583.
[http://dx.doi.org/10.1557/JMR.1992.1564]

[17]   Manzur, T.; Yazdani, N.; Emon, M.A.B. Potential of Carbon Nanotube Reinforced Cement Composites as Concrete Repair Material. *J. Nanomater.,* **2016**, *2016*, 1-10.
[http://dx.doi.org/10.1155/2016/1421959]

[18]   Tonelli, M.; Baglioni, P.; Ridi, F. Halloysite Nanotubes as Nano-Carriers of Corrosion Inhibitors in Cement Formulations. *Materials (Basel),* **2020**, *13*(14), 3150.
[http://dx.doi.org/10.3390/ma13143150] [PMID: 32679758]

[19]   ERŞAN, Y. Ç. Self-healing performance of biogranule containing microbial self-healing concrete under intermittent Wet/Dry cycles. *Journal of Polytechnic,* **2020**.
[http://dx.doi.org/10.2339/politeknik.742210]

[20]   ZHANG, L.; WANG, W.; YU, D. Self-healing cellulose membranes prepared by microcapsules containing uv-initiated healing agents. *DEStech Transactions on Materials Science and Engineering,* **2017**.
[http://dx.doi.org/10.12783/dtmse/amsee2017/14249]

[21]   Rajczakowska, M.; Habermehl-Cwirzen, K.; Hedlund, H.; Cwirzen, A. Autogenous Self-Healing: A Better Solution for Concrete. *J. Mater. Civ. Eng.,* **2019**, *31*(9), 03119001.
[http://dx.doi.org/10.1061/(ASCE)MT.1943-5533.0002764]

[22]   Sanchez, F.; Sobolev, K. Nanotechnology in concrete – A review. *Constr. Build. Mater.,* **2010**, *24*(11), 2060-2071.
[http://dx.doi.org/10.1016/j.conbuildmat.2010.03.014]

[23]   Duncan, T.V. Applications of nanotechnology in food packaging and food safety: Barrier materials, antimicrobials and sensors. *J. Colloid Interface Sci.,* **2011**, *363*(1), 1-24.
[http://dx.doi.org/10.1016/j.jcis.2011.07.017] [PMID: 21824625]

[24]   De Belie, N.; Gruyaert, E.; Al-Tabbaa, A.; Antonaci, P.; Baera, C.; Bajare, D.; Darquennes, A.; Davies, R.; Ferrara, L.; Jefferson, T.; Litina, C.; Miljevic, B.; Otlewska, A.; Ranogajec, J.; Roig-Flores, M.; Paine, K.; Lukowski, P.; Serna, P.; Tulliani, J.M.; Vucetic, S.; Wang, J.; Jonkers, H.M. A Review of Self-Healing Concrete for Damage Management of Structures. *Adv. Mater. Interfaces,* **2018**, *5*(17), 1800074.
[http://dx.doi.org/10.1002/admi.201800074]

[25]   Blaiszik, B.J.; Kramer, S.L.B.; Olugebefola, S.C.; Moore, J.S.; Sottos, N.R.; White, S.R. Self-Healing Polymers and Composites. *Annu. Rev. Mater. Res.,* **2010**, *40*(1), 179-211.
[http://dx.doi.org/10.1146/annurev-matsci-070909-104532]

[26]   Yang, F.; Siahkouhi, M.; Liu, G. A Study on possibility of application of recent self-healing methods for self-healing concrete railway sleeper manufacturing: a review. *Acta Polytech. Hung.,* **2024**, *21*(1), 135-152.
[http://dx.doi.org/10.12700/APH.21.1.2024.1.9]

[27]   Ahn, T.H.; Kishi, T. Crack Self-healing Behavior of Cementitious Composites Incorporating Various Mineral Admixtures. *J. Adv. Concr. Technol.,* **2010**, *8*(2), 171-186.
[http://dx.doi.org/10.3151/jact.8.171]

[28]   De Muynck, W.; De Belie, N.; Verstraete, W. Microbial carbonate precipitation in construction materials: A review. *Ecol. Eng.,* **2010**, *36*(2), 118-136.
[http://dx.doi.org/10.1016/j.ecoleng.2009.02.006]

[29]   Lloyd, S.M.; Lave, L.B.; Matthews, H.S. Life cycle benefits of using nanotechnology to stabilize platinum-group metal particles in automotive catalysts. *Environ. Sci. Technol.,* **2005**, *39*(5), 1384-1392.
[http://dx.doi.org/10.1021/es049325w] [PMID: 15787381]

[30]   Marinelli, A.; Diamanti, M.V.; Lucotti, A.; Pedeferri, M.P.; Del Curto, B. Evaluation of Coatings to Improve the Durability and Water-Barrier Properties of Corrugated Cardboard. *Coatings,* **2021**, *12*(1), 10.

[http://dx.doi.org/10.3390/coatings12010010]

[31]   Wu, S.; Xiong, G.; Yang, H.; Gong, B.; Tian, Y.; Xu, C.; Wang, Y.; Fisher, T.S.; Yan, J.; Cen, K.; Luo, T.; Tu, X.; Bo, Z. Kostya Ostrikov. *Multifunctional Solar Waterways: Plasma-Enabled Self-Cleaning Nanoarchitectures for Energy-Efficient Desalination.*, **2019**, *9*(30), 1901286-1901286. [http://dx.doi.org/10.1002/aenm.201901286]

[32]   Camargo, P.H.C.; Satyanarayana, K.G.; Wypych, F. Nanocomposites: synthesis, structure, properties and new application opportunities. *Mater. Res.*, **2009**, *12*(1), 1-39. [http://dx.doi.org/10.1590/S1516-14392009000100002]

[33]   Moulder, D.S. Impacts of construction activities in wetlands of the United States. *Mar. Pollut. Bull.*, **1977**, *8*(3), 71. [http://dx.doi.org/10.1016/0025-326X(77)90252-1]

[34]   Sharma, V.K.; Yngard, R.A.; Lin, Y. Silver nanoparticles: Green synthesis and their antimicrobial activities. *Adv. Colloid Interface Sci.*, **2009**, *145*(1-2), 83-96. [http://dx.doi.org/10.1016/j.cis.2008.09.002] [PMID: 18945421]

[35]   Srinivas, P.; Patra, C.R.; Bhattacharya, S.; Mukhopadhyay, D. Cytotoxicity of naphthoquinones and their capacity to generate reactive oxygen species is quenched when conjugated with gold nanoparticles. *Int. J. Nanomedicine*, **2011**, *6*, 2113-2122. [http://dx.doi.org/10.2147/IJN.S24074] [PMID: 22114475]

[36]   Sharma, S.; Alam, M.A.; Sharma, A.; Singh, P.; Dhoundiyal, S.; Sharma, A. High-Impact Applications of IoT System-Based Metaheuristics. In: *Nature-Inspired Methods for Smart Healthcare Systems and Medical Data*; Springer Nature: Switzerland, **2023**; pp. 121-131.

[37]   Krishnamoorti, R. Technology Tomorrow: Extracting the Benefits of Nanotechnology for the Oil Industry. *J. Pet. Technol.*, **2006**, *58*(11), 24-26. [http://dx.doi.org/10.2118/1106-0024-JPT]

[38]   Gordon, R.; Sinton, D.; Kavanagh, K.L.; Brolo, A.G. A new generation of sensors based on extraordinary optical transmission. *Acc. Chem. Res.*, **2008**, *41*(8), 1049-1057. [http://dx.doi.org/10.1021/ar800074d] [PMID: 18605739]

[39]   Epps, R.W.; Volk, A.A. Malek; Milad Abolhasani. Universal Self-Driving Laboratory for Accelerated Discovery of Materials and Molecules. *Chem*, **2021**, *7*(10), 2541-2545. [http://dx.doi.org/10.1016/j.chempr.2021.09.004]

[40]   Seager, T.P.; Linkov, I. Coupling Multicriteria Decision Analysis and Life Cycle Assessment for Nanomaterials. *J. Ind. Ecol.*, **2008**, *12*(3), 282-285. [http://dx.doi.org/10.1111/j.1530-9290.2008.00048.x]

[41]   Gao, Z. Overall design of cable-stayed bridge for main channel bridge of Donghai Bridge. *Prestress Technology*, **2011**, *15*(2), 3-19. [http://dx.doi.org/10.59238/j.pt.2011.02.001]

[42]   Senar, J.C.; Domènech, J.; Arroyo, L.; Torre, I.; Gordo, D. An evaluation of monk parakeet damage to crops in the metropolitan area of Barcelona. *Anim. Biodivers. Conserv.*, **2016**, *39*(1), 141-145. [http://dx.doi.org/10.32800/abc.2016.39.0141]

[43]   Randeree, K.; Ahmed, N. The social imperative in sustainable urban development. *Smart and Sustainable Built Environment*, **2019**, *8*(2), 138-149. [http://dx.doi.org/10.1108/SASBE-11-2017-0064]

[44]   Warshawsky, D.N. The devolution of urban food waste governance: Case study of food rescue in Los Angeles. *Cities*, **2015**, *49*, 26-34. [http://dx.doi.org/10.1016/j.cities.2015.06.006]

[45]   Zhang, H.; Liu, H.; Tian, Z-Q. Dylan Dah-Chuan Lu; Yu, Y.; Stefano Cestellos-Blanco; Sakimoto, K. K.; Yang, P. *Bacteria Photosensitized by Intracellular Gold Nanoclusters for Solar Fuel Production.*, **2018**, *13*(10), 900-905.

[http://dx.doi.org/10.1038/s41565-018-0267-z] [PMID: 30275495]

[46]   Labaran, Y.H.; Atmaca, N.; Tan, M.; Atmaca, K.; Aram, S.A.; Kaky, A.T. Nano-enhanced concrete: unveiling the impact of nano-silica on strength, durability, and cost efficiency. *Discover Civil Engineering,* **2024**, *1*(1), 116.
[http://dx.doi.org/10.1007/s44290-024-00120-9]

[47]   Caruso, F. Nanoengineering of Particle Surfaces. *Adv. Mater.,* **2001**, *13*(1), 11-22.
[http://dx.doi.org/10.1002/1521-4095(200101)13:1<11::AID-ADMA11>3.0.CO;2-N]

[48]   Mittal, D.; Kaur, G.; Singh, P.; Yadav, K.; Ali, S.A. Nanoparticle-Based Sustainable Agriculture and Food Science: Recent Advances and Future Outlook. *Frontiers in Nanotechnology,* **2020**, *2*, 579954.
[http://dx.doi.org/10.3389/fnano.2020.579954]

[49]   Zhao, Y.; Jiang, L. Hollow Micro/Nanomaterials with Multilevel Interior Structures. *Adv. Mater.,* **2009**, *21*(36), 3621-3638.
[http://dx.doi.org/10.1002/adma.200803645]

[50]   Batley, G.E.; Kirby, J.K.; McLaughlin, M.J. Fate and risks of nanomaterials in aquatic and terrestrial environments. *Acc. Chem. Res.,* **2013**, *46*(3), 854-862.
[http://dx.doi.org/10.1021/ar2003368] [PMID: 22759090]

[51]   Loveridge, D.; Dewick, P.; Randles, S. Converging technologies at the nanoscale: The making of a new world? *Technol. Anal. Strateg. Manage.,* **2008**, *20*(1), 29-43.
[http://dx.doi.org/10.1080/09537320701726544]

[52]   Turner, B. *International Organization for Standardization*; ISO, **2003**, pp. 47-47.

[53]   Fisher, E. The 'perfect storm' of REACH: charting regulatory controversy in the age of information, sustainable development, and globalization. *J. Risk Res.,* **2008**, *11*(4), 541-563.
[http://dx.doi.org/10.1080/13669870802086547]

[54]   Oberdörster, G.; Oberdörster, E.; Oberdörster, J. Nanotoxicology: an emerging discipline evolving from studies of ultrafine particles. *Environ. Health Perspect.,* **2005**, *113*(7), 823-839.
[http://dx.doi.org/10.1289/ehp.7339] [PMID: 16002369]

[55]   Schrand, A.M.; Huang, H.; Carlson, C.; Schlager, J.J.; Ōsawa, E.; Hussain, S.M.; Dai, L. Are diamond nanoparticles cytotoxic? *J. Phys. Chem. B,* **2007**, *111*(1), 2-7.
[http://dx.doi.org/10.1021/jp066387v] [PMID: 17201422]

CHAPTER 5

Nanoelectronics and Quantum Frontier

Abstract: This chapter investigates the rapidly advancing fields of nanoelectronics and quantum computing, two domains at the forefront of modern technology. Nanoelectronics, a subfield of nanotechnology, involves manipulating materials at the nanoscale to create electronic components with enhanced performance, efficiency, and functionality. The chapter begins by defining nanoelectronics, tracing its historical development, and highlighting its significance in various industries, from consumer electronics to telecommunications. It then explores the fundamental principles of nanoelectronics, focusing on nanoscale effects, electronic transport, and the unique properties of nanomaterials. Moving beyond the basics, the chapter discusses the latest developments in nanoelectronic devices, including nanoscale transistors like FinFETs and Tunnel FETs, as well as emerging technologies like single-electron transistors and spintronics devices. The integration of quantum dots, which offer remarkable quantum confinement effects, is examined in the context of nanoelectronics, along with their fabrication techniques and applications. The chapter also introduces the fundamentals of quantum computing, explaining the concept of qubits, superposition, and quantum entanglement, which enable quantum computers to solve complex problems that are intractable for classical computers. The potential advantages and challenges of both nanoelectronics and quantum computing are explored, including manufacturing difficulties, heat dissipation issues, and ethical considerations. Finally, the chapter looks to the future, discussing emerging trends in nanoelectronics, the trajectory of quantum computing, and the broader implications for industry and society. Together, these advancements promise to revolutionize technology and bring transformative changes to a wide range of fields.

Keywords: Electronic transport, Nanoelectronics, Nanoscale transistors, Quantum dots, Quantum computing, Quantum entanglement, Size-dependent properties.

INTRODUCTION

Nanoelectronics is a branch of electronics that deals with electronic components, systems, and devices at the nanoscale, typically less than 100 nanometers in size. This field leverages the unique properties of nanomaterials and quantum mechanical phenomena to design and develop innovative technologies. At the nanoscale, electrons behave differently due to quantum effects, leading to new

Shivang Dhoundiyal & Aftab Alam

opportunities for manipulating electronic properties [1]. Nanoelectronics encompasses a broad range of devices and applications, including transistors, sensors, memory devices, and logic gates, all of which are integral to advanced computing systems, energy-efficient devices, and next-generation communication technologies. The scope of nanoelectronics is vast, with potential applications in fields as diverse as medicine, energy, consumer electronics, and even quantum computing, positioning it as a cornerstone of future technological advancements.

The development of nanoelectronics is deeply intertwined with the evolution of semiconductor technology. The journey began with the invention of the transistor in 1947 by Bell Labs, which paved the way for modern electronics [2]. As transistor sizes shrank over the decades, the industry adhered to Moore's Law, predicting the doubling of transistors on a chip approximately every two years. This trend continued until the dimensions of electronic components approached the nanoscale in the early 21st century. The transition to nanoelectronics was marked by significant milestones, such as the development of FinFET (Fin Field-Effect Transistor) technology and the rise of nanomaterials like graphene and carbon nanotubes [3]. These advancements enabled the creation of smaller, faster, and more efficient electronic devices. Historical breakthroughs in quantum mechanics and materials science further enriched the field, allowing researchers to explore new paradigms like quantum dots and molecular electronics. The development of nanoelectronics reflects a continuous effort to push the boundaries of miniaturization and performance in electronics, as mentioned in Table **5.1**.

Nanoelectronics plays a critical role in shaping modern technology. The shrinking of electronic components to the nanoscale has led to unprecedented improvements in performance, energy efficiency, and integration density. This has enabled the creation of powerful processors, compact storage devices, and energy-efficient systems that drive everything from smartphones and laptops to advanced medical devices and autonomous vehicles. Nanoelectronics is also at the heart of emerging technologies like the Internet of Things (IoT), where billions of interconnected devices require ultra-small, low-power electronics to function seamlessly [4]. Nanoelectronics is foundational to the development of quantum computing, a revolutionary technology that promises to solve complex problems beyond the reach of classical computers. The impact of nanoelectronics extends to various industries, including healthcare, where nanoscale sensors and devices enable early disease detection and targeted drug delivery, as depicted in Fig. (**5.1**). Nanoelectronics contributes to the efficiency of solar cells and energy storage systems in renewable energy. As technology continues to evolve, the importance of nanoelectronics will only grow, driving innovations that redefine how we live, work, and interact with the world.

Table 5.1. Overview of nanoelectronics and quantum computing.

Aspect	Nanoelectronics	Quantum Computing	References
Definition	Study and application of electronic components at the nanoscale for improved performance and efficiency.	Use of quantum-mechanical phenomena to perform computations that surpass classical computing capabilities.	[5]
Key Technologies	Nanoscale Transistors (*e.g.*, FinFETs, Tunnel FETs)	Quantum Bits (Qubits)	[6]
-	Nano-MOSFETs	Quantum Gates	[7]
-	Spintronics devices	Quantum algorithms	[8]
Core principles	Quantum confinement	Superposition and entanglement	[9]
-	Tunneling	Quantum interference	[10]
-	Size-dependent properties	Quantum parallelism	[11]
Applications	High-performance computing	Cryptography and secure communications	[12]
-	Wearable electronics	Drug discovery and material science	[13]
-	Energy-efficient devices	Optimization problems	[14]
Fabrication techniques	Lithography	Qubit fabrication (*e.g.*, superconducting qubits, trapped ions)	[15]
-	Self-assembly	Quantum circuit design	[16]
-	Atomic layer deposition	Error correction methods	[17]
Advantages	Miniaturization of devices	Exponential speedup for certain problems	[18]
-	Enhanced energy efficiency	Solving classically intractable problems	[19]
-	Faster processing speeds	Potential to revolutionize industries	[20]
Challenges	Manufacturing scalability	Quantum decoherence and error correction	[21]
-	Heat dissipation	Hardware stability	[22]
-	Power consumption issues	Complex algorithm development	[23]
Future directions	Integration with iot and smart devices	Development of fault-tolerant quantum computers	[24]
-	2d materials (*e.g.*, graphene)	Exploration of new qubit technologies	[25]
-	Neuromorphic computing	Quantum cryptography and quantum networks	[26]
Ethical and Security Considerations	Environmental impact of nanomaterial production	Data privacy and security risks	[27]

(Table 5.1) cont.....

Aspect	Nanoelectronics	Quantum Computing	References
-	Potential for widening the digital divide	Ethical implications of quantum supremacy	[28]
-	Regulatory challenges	Equity in access to quantum technologies	[29]

Nanochip Delivery System for the Treatment of Brain Disorders

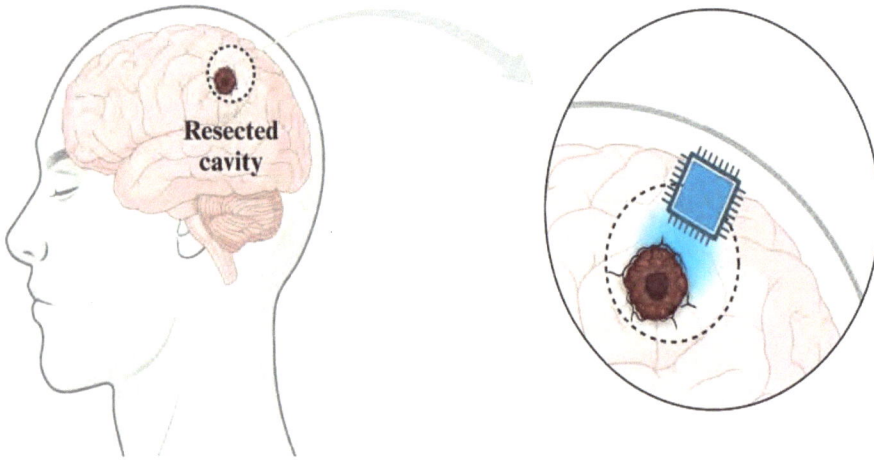

Fig. (5.1). Role of nanoelectronics in healthcare systems.

BASICS OF NANOELECTRONICS

At the nanoscale, materials and devices exhibit unique physical and chemical properties that differ significantly from their bulk counterparts. This is largely due to the increased surface area-to-volume ratio, quantum mechanical effects, and the dominance of surface forces over bulk properties. Nanoscale effects influence various parameters such as electrical conductivity, optical properties, and mechanical strength. In nanoelectronics, the behavior of electrons is governed by quantum mechanics rather than classical physics, leading to phenomena like quantum confinement and tunneling [30]. These effects become critical when the dimensions of a material or device are reduced to the nanometer scale, where traditional assumptions about electrical behavior no longer hold. Understanding these effects is essential for designing and optimizing nanoscale electronic devices, as they can lead to enhanced performance, lower power consumption, and new functionalities not possible at larger scales.

In nanoelectronics, electronic transport refers to the movement of electrons through nanoscale materials and devices. At this scale, transport mechanisms differ from those in larger structures due to quantum effects and reduced dimensionality. In nanostructures like quantum dots, nanowires, and thin films, electrons can experience phenomena such as ballistic transport, where they move through the material without scattering, or quantum tunneling, where they pass through energy barriers they could not overcome in larger structures [31]. These mechanisms lead to significant changes in conductivity and resistivity, making electronic transport in nanostructures a key factor in device design. Understanding these transport properties allows researchers to engineer nanoscale devices with improved speed, efficiency, and precision, enabling applications in areas such as high-performance computing and low-power electronics.

Quantum tunneling and confinement are two fundamental phenomena that arise at the nanoscale and are central to nanoelectronics. Quantum tunneling occurs when electrons pass through energy barriers that would be insurmountable in classical physics, enabling the creation of ultra-thin transistors and tunnel diodes. This effect is crucial for devices like the tunnel field-effect transistor (TFET), which promises to reduce power consumption in future electronic devices [32]. Quantum confinement, on the other hand, occurs when the dimensions of a material are reduced to the point where the motion of electrons is restricted, typically in one or more directions. This confinement leads to discrete energy levels, altering the electronic and optical properties of the material. Quantum dots, for example, exhibit size-dependent light emission due to quantum confinement. Both tunneling and quantum confinement enable the design of nanoscale devices with unique properties, paving the way for innovations in transistors, sensors, and memory devices [33].

One of the defining features of nanomaterials is that their properties are highly dependent on size. As materials are reduced to the nanoscale, they can exhibit changes in electronic, optical, thermal, and mechanical properties. The electrical conductivity of a nanomaterial can increase or decrease depending on its size, shape, and surface characteristics. Similarly, the optical properties of nanoparticles can vary, leading to phenomena such as surface plasmon resonance, which is used in sensing applications. The mechanical properties of nanomaterials, such as strength and flexibility, also change at the nanoscale, enabling the development of lightweight and durable materials [34]. Understanding and controlling these size-dependent properties are crucial in nanoelectronics, as this allows for tailoring materials and devices to achieve specific performance characteristics. This has far-reaching implications in areas such as flexible electronics, photonics, and energy storage, where the ability to fine-tune material properties is essential for innovation.

PRINCIPLES AND DEVICES

Nanoelectronics is built upon several fundamental concepts that distinguish it from traditional electronics. One of the key ideas is the influence of quantum mechanics on the behavior of electrons at the nanoscale. Unlike classical electronics, where electron behavior is predictable and governed by established physical laws, nanoelectronics operates in a realm where quantum effects dominate. This includes phenomena such as quantum confinement, tunneling, and discrete energy levels. Another important concept is the role of nanomaterials, which possess unique electrical, optical, and mechanical properties that can be tuned by manipulating their size, shape, and structure [35]. Additionally, nanoelectronics explores the use of alternative charge carriers, such as spin in spintronics, as opposed to just the traditional electron flow. These concepts collectively enable the creation of devices that are smaller, faster, more energy-efficient, and capable of performing new functions, thus expanding the possibilities of electronic technology.

Nanoscale transistors are the cornerstone of modern nanoelectronics. New transistor architectures have emerged as traditional MOSFETs (Metal-Oxide-emiconductor Field-Effect Transistors) approach their physical limits due to scaling challenges. FinFETs (Fin Field-Effect Transistors) are a prime example of this innovation. FinFETs use a three-dimensional structure where the conducting channel is elevated above the substrate in a fin-like shape [36]. This design provides better control over the channel, reducing leakage currents and allowing for faster switching speeds, which are crucial for high-performance processors. Another important nanoscale transistor is the Tunnel FET (TFET), which leverages quantum tunneling to achieve extremely low power consumption. Unlike traditional transistors, which require a threshold voltage to switch on and off, TFETs allow current to flow even at lower voltages, making them ideal for ultra-low-power applications [37]. These nanoscale transistors represent significant advancements in electronics, enabling continued performance improvements in computing, communication, and energy-efficient devices.

Nano-MOSFETs (Metal-Oxide-Semiconductor Field-Effect Transistors) are scaled-down versions of conventional MOSFETs, designed to operate efficiently at the nanoscale. As the size of transistors shrinks, nano-MOSFETs face challenges such as short-channel effects, increased leakage currents, and variability in performance [38]. To address these issues, new materials such as high-k dielectrics and metal gates have been introduced, along with novel device architectures like FinFETs. Nano-MOSFETs are integral to modern integrated circuits, forming the building blocks of microprocessors, memory chips, and digital logic circuits. Their applications span a wide range of fields, from consumer electronics to telecommunications, automotive systems, and industrial automation [39]. In the medical field, nano-MOSFETs are used in biosensors and medical imaging devices. In energy applications, they enable efficient power management in renewable energy systems and electric vehicles. The continued development of nano-MOSFETs is critical for advancing the capabilities of electronic devices and systems.

Beyond transistors, a variety of other nanoelectronic devices are being developed to harness the unique properties of nanomaterials and quantum effects. One such device is the Single-Electron Transistor (SET), which operates by controlling the flow of individual electrons through a nanoscale island [40]. SETs offer high sensitivity and low power consumption, making them suitable for applications in precision measurement and quantum computing. Another emerging area is spintronics, which exploits the intrinsic spin of electrons, in addition to their charge, to store and process information. Spintronic devices, such as magnetic tunnel junctions and spin valves, offer advantages like non-volatility, faster switching speeds, and lower energy consumption compared to traditional electronics. These devices are already being used in applications such as magnetic random-access memory (MRAM) and advanced sensors [41]. The development of these and other nanoelectronic devices holds the potential to revolutionize electronics, offering new functionalities and efficiencies that go beyond what is possible with conventional technologies.

QUANTUM DOTS AND TRANSISTORS

Quantum dots (QDs) are nanoscale semiconductor particles that exhibit distinct quantum mechanical properties due to their size, which typically ranges from 2 to 10 nanometers [42]. These tiny structures have electronic properties that are significantly different from bulk materials due to quantum confinement, where the electrons are restricted in all three spatial dimensions. As a result, quantum dots have discrete energy levels, similar to those of atoms, which is why they are sometimes referred to as "artificial atoms." This unique behavior enables quantum dots to absorb and emit light at specific wavelengths, which can be precisely tuned by changing the size of the quantum dot. Smaller quantum dots emit higher-energy light (blue), while larger ones emit lower-energy light (red) [43]. This size-dependent tunability of optical properties makes quantum dots invaluable in applications such as display technology, where they enhance color accuracy and brightness in quantum dot displays (QLEDs) [44]. In addition to their optical properties, quantum dots also exhibit unique electrical characteristics, making them suitable for applications in nanoelectronics, including transistors and photodetectors. Their ability to operate at low power and their potential for integration into various materials have positioned quantum dots at the forefront of nanoscale device innovation. The fabrication of quantum dots involves several sophisticated techniques, each offering control over the size, shape, and composition of the dots, which are crucial for their functionality. One of the most widely used methods is colloidal synthesis, where quantum dots are created in a liquid medium by reacting precursor materials in the presence of surfactants. This method allows for large-scale production and precise control over the size and surface properties of the quantum dots, making it popular for commercial applications in displays and solar cells. Another important method is molecular beam epitaxy (MBE), a high-precision technique where quantum dots are grown layer by layer on a substrate in an ultra-high vacuum environment. MBE is particularly useful for creating high-quality quantum dots integrated into solid-state devices, such as quantum dot lasers and infrared detectors. Chemical vapor deposition (CVD) is another technique, often used for creating quantum dots from materials like silicon and carbon. In addition, lithographic techniques, such as electron-beam lithography, allow for the precise patterning of quantum dots on semiconductor surfaces, enabling their integration into complex electronic circuits [45]. Each fabrication technique has its advantages and trade-offs, with researchers continually refining these processes to achieve better control over the properties of quantum dots. For example, colloidal synthesis offers scalability and tunable properties, making it ideal for applications in consumer electronics, while techniques like molecular beam epitaxy (MBE) and chemical vapor deposition (CVD) provide high precision and integration capabilities for more specialized devices. Advances in quantum dot fabrication are crucial for pushing the boundaries of nanoelectronics, enabling the creation of devices with enhanced performance and novel functionalities.

Quantum dot-based transistors represent a significant leap in transistor technology, leveraging the unique properties of quantum dots to achieve enhanced functionality at the nanoscale. These transistors operate by using quantum dots as the active elements in the channel, where the behavior of electrons is controlled by quantum confinement. This allows for precise manipulation of electronic states and enables the transistor to switch between on and off states with minimal energy loss. One of the most promising types of quantum dot transistors is the Single-Electron Transistor (SET), where the flow of individual electrons through the quantum dot is controlled by a gate voltage [46]. SETs exhibit extremely low power consumption and high sensitivity, making them ideal for applications in quantum computing, where they can serve as qubits, the fundamental units of quantum information, as depicted in Fig. (**5.2**). In addition to SETs, quantum dots are being integrated into more traditional transistor designs, such as Quantum Dot Field-Effect Transistors (QDFETs), which offer enhanced performance in terms of speed, efficiency, and scaling. These transistors are being explored for use in next-generation logic circuits, memory devices, and sensors, where their unique properties can provide advantages over conventional semiconductor technologies.

Another exciting area of research is the use of quantum dots in flexible and transparent electronics. By incorporating quantum dots into flexible substrates, researchers are developing transistors that can bend and stretch while maintaining their performance. This opens up possibilities for wearable electronics, foldable displays, and other innovative applications. Quantum dot-based transistors are also being studied for their potential in energy-harvesting devices, where they can convert light or heat into electrical energy with high efficiency. As research in this field progresses, quantum dot transistors are expected to play a crucial role in the future of nanoelectronics, enabling the development of smaller, faster, and more energy-efficient devices. Quantum dots have a wide range of applications in nanoelectronics, thanks to their unique optical and electronic properties. One of the most prominent applications is in display technology, where quantum dots are used in Quantum Dot Light-Emitting Diodes (QD-LEDs) and Quantum Dot Displays (QLEDs) [47]. These displays offer superior color accuracy, brightness, and energy efficiency compared to traditional LCD and OLED displays. Quantum dots are also being integrated into solar cells, where their ability to absorb and convert sunlight into electricity can significantly improve the efficiency of photovoltaic devices. By tuning the size of the quantum dots, researchers can optimize the absorption spectrum of the solar cell, allowing it to capture a broader range of sunlight. In addition to optoelectronics, quantum dots are making an impact on memory devices. Quantum dot flash memory, for example, uses quantum dots as charge storage elements, enabling higher data storage densities and faster read/write speeds compared to conventional flash memory. Quantum dots are also being explored for use in quantum computing, where their discrete energy levels and ability to entangle electrons make them ideal candidates for qubits [48]. In quantum sensors, quantum dots can detect minute changes in light, temperature, or magnetic fields, making them useful for applications in medical diagnostics, environmental monitoring, and security systems. Beyond traditional electronics, quantum dots are finding applications in biomedicine, where they are used as fluorescent markers for imaging and diagnostics. Their bright, stable light emission makes them ideal for tracking biological processes in real-time. In addition, quantum dots are being explored for drug delivery, where their small size and ability to penetrate biological barriers can be used to target specific cells or tissues with therapeutic agents [49].

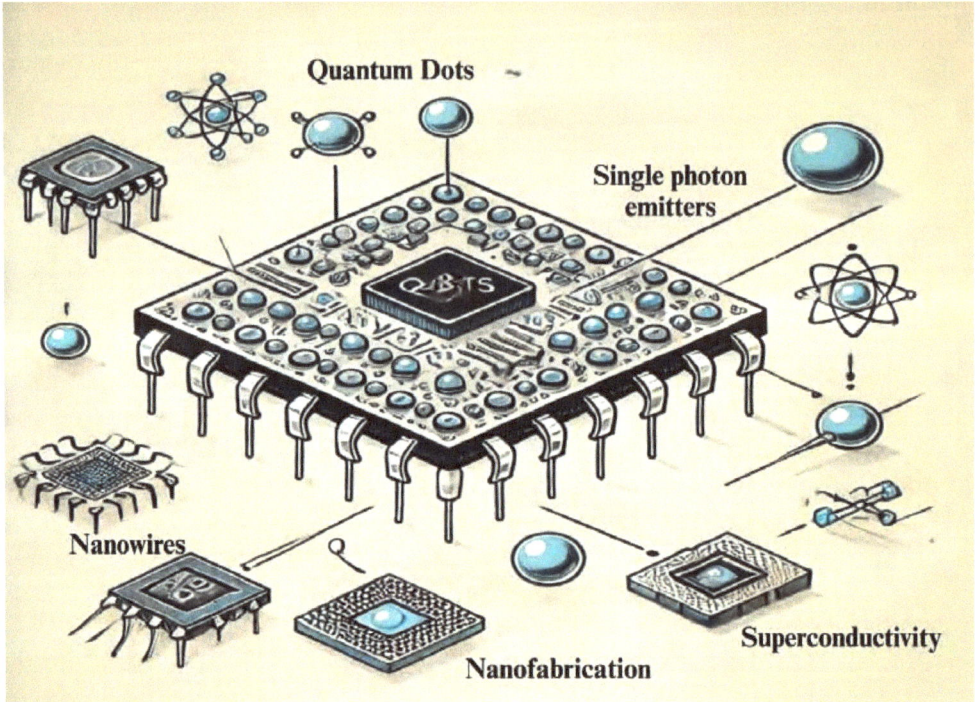

Fig. (5.2). Applications of nanotechnology in quantum electronics.

QUANTUM COMPUTING

Quantum computing is a cutting-edge field of computing that leverages the principles of quantum mechanics to perform complex calculations far beyond the capabilities of classical computers. Unlike classical computers, which use binary bits (0s and 1s) as the fundamental units of information, quantum computers use quantum bits, or qubits, which can exist in multiple states simultaneously [50]. This allows quantum computers to process a vast amount of information in parallel, making them exponentially more powerful for certain tasks. The potential of quantum computing lies in its ability to solve problems that are currently intractable for classical computers, such as simulating complex molecules, optimizing large systems, and breaking cryptographic codes. As research in this field advances, quantum computing is expected to revolutionize industries such as pharmaceuticals, finance, logistics, and cybersecurity. Quantum computing is built on the principles of quantum mechanics, a branch of physics that describes the behavior of matter and energy at the atomic and subatomic levels. Key quantum phenomena, such as superposition and entanglement, enable quantum computers to perform operations in ways that are fundamentally different from classical computers. While still in the experimental stage, quantum computers have already demonstrated their potential in tasks like factoring large numbers, solving linear equations, and simulating quantum systems. Companies like IBM, Google, and Microsoft, as well as various research institutions, are actively working on developing quantum computing hardware and software, pushing the boundaries of what is possible in the world of computation [51]. Qubits are the basic units of information in a quantum computer, analogous to classical bits in traditional computers. However, unlike classical bits, which can only represent a state of 0 or 1, qubits can exist in a superposition of both states simultaneously. This means that a qubit can represent 0, 1, or any quantum combination of these states. Superposition is a key feature of quantum computing, as it allows quantum computers to process multiple possibilities at once, vastly increasing their computational power. For example, while a classical computer with n bits can represent only one of 2^n possible states at a time, a quantum computer with n qubits can represent all 2^n states simultaneously [52]. Superposition is typically achieved in physical systems like atoms, ions, or superconducting circuits, which are carefully manipulated using lasers, microwaves, or magnetic fields. These qubits are maintained in their superposition state until a measurement is made, at which point the superposition collapses to a definite state of 0 or 1. The ability to maintain and manipulate qubits in superposition is a key challenge in quantum computing, as qubits are highly sensitive to environmental noise and can easily lose their quantum properties, a phenomenon known as decoherence. Researchers are actively exploring different qubit technologies, such as trapped ions, superconducting circuits, and topological qubits, to develop more stable and scalable quantum computers. Quantum entanglement is another fundamental concept in quantum computing, where the states of two or more qubits become linked in such a way that the state of one qubit directly affects the state of the other, regardless of the distance between them. This phenomenon, described by Albert Einstein as "spooky action at a distance," allows entangled qubits to share information instantaneously [53]. Entanglement is a crucial resource in quantum computing, enabling the creation of complex quantum states and the performance of quantum operations that are impossible with classical systems. Entangled qubits can be used to implement quantum gates, which are the building blocks of quantum circuits. Quantum gates, like their classical counterparts, perform operations on qubits, but they exploit the unique properties of quantum mechanics. For example, the Hadamard gate creates a superposition state, while the CNOT (Controlled-NOT) gate creates entanglement between qubits. Unlike classical gates, which operate on individual bits, quantum gates can manipulate the states of multiple qubits simultaneously, allowing for complex quantum operations. Quantum circuits, composed of sequences of quantum gates, are used to implement quantum algorithms that solve specific problems. One of the most famous examples of a quantum gate is the quantum Fourier transform, which is essential in algorithms for factoring large numbers and searching databases [54]. The implementation of quantum gates requires precise control over qubits and their interactions, making hardware design a significant challenge in quantum computing. As quantum technology advances, researchers are working to develop more efficient and error-resistant quantum gates, paving the way for more powerful quantum computers.

Quantum algorithms are the instructions that quantum computers follow to solve specific problems. Unlike classical algorithms, which rely on step-by-step logical operations, quantum algorithms leverage quantum phenomena such as superposition, entanglement, and interference to achieve results that are impossible or impractical for classical computers. Some of the most well-known quantum algorithms include Shor's algorithm for factoring large numbers, Grover's algorithm for searching unsorted databases, and the quantum simulation algorithm for modeling quantum systems. Shor's algorithm is particularly significant because it can factor large integers exponentially faster than the best-known classical algorithms. This poses a potential threat to current cryptographic systems, which rely on the difficulty of factoring large numbers for security [55]. Grover's algorithm, on the other hand, provides a quadratic speedup for unstructured search problems, making it valuable for a wide range of applications, from database search to optimization problems. Quantum simulation algorithms are another key application of quantum computing, enabling the simulation of complex quantum systems that are beyond the reach of classical computers. This has profound implications for fields such as chemistry, materials science, and drug discovery, where accurate simulations of molecular interactions and quantum phenomena are crucial. For example, quantum computers could help design new materials with specific properties, optimize chemical reactions for energy efficiency, or discover new drugs by simulating the interactions between molecules and proteins. Potential future applications include machine learning, artificial intelligence, optimization of complex systems (such as supply chains or financial portfolios), and solving differential equations in physics and engineering, represented in Fig. (**5.3**). The ability of quantum computers to handle vast amounts of data and perform complex calculations in parallel offers the promise of breakthroughs in areas that are currently limited by classical computing capabilities.

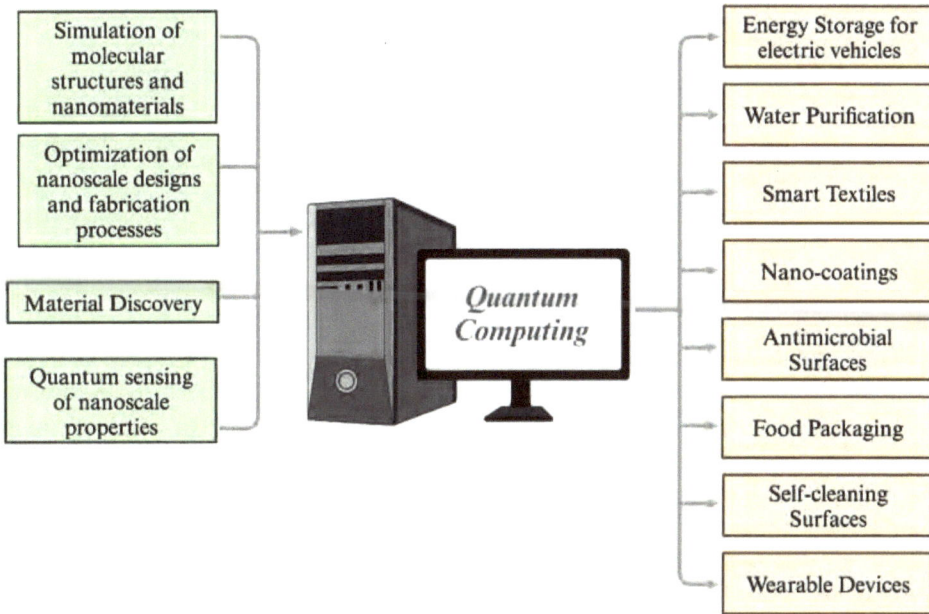

Fig. (5.3). Role of quantum computing in varied fields of nanotechnologies.

POTENTIAL AND CHALLENGES

Nanoelectronics and quantum computing offer transformative advantages over traditional technologies, promising to revolutionize industries ranging from computing to healthcare. Nanoelectronics, by exploiting the unique properties of materials at the nanoscale, enables the creation of devices that are smaller, faster, and more efficient than conventional electronics. These advances lead to more powerful and compact processors, memory devices with higher storage capacities, and sensors with enhanced sensitivity. For instance, nanoelectronics has the potential to extend Moore's Law, allowing for the continuous miniaturization of transistors and other components in integrated circuits [56]. In consumer electronics, this translates into more powerful smartphones, longer-lasting batteries, and enhanced user experiences with faster processing speeds and better graphics. Quantum computing, on the other hand, represents a paradigm shift in how we approach complex problem-solving. Unlike classical computers, which process information sequentially, quantum computers leverage superposition and entanglement to perform multiple calculations simultaneously. This capability makes quantum computers exponentially faster at solving certain types of problems, such as factoring large numbers (which has implications for cryptography), simulating quantum systems (which is vital for drug discovery and materials science), and optimizing large-scale systems (such as supply chains and financial portfolios) [57]. The potential applications of quantum computing are vast, ranging from breaking current encryption methods to designing new molecules for pharmaceuticals to solving complex optimization problems that are currently intractable for classical computers. Additionally, quantum computing's ability to simulate quantum systems accurately can lead to breakthroughs in understanding fundamental physics, chemistry, and biology. This could pave the way for innovations in renewable energy, new materials, and medical treatments. Despite their potential, nanoelectronics and quantum computing face significant challenges in manufacturing and scalability. In nanoelectronics, the miniaturization of components to the nanoscale introduces difficulties in fabrication and assembly. Traditional lithography techniques used in semiconductor manufacturing are approaching their physical limits, making it increasingly challenging to create smaller and more densely packed transistors. Additionally, variations at the nanoscale, such as defects in materials or fluctuations in the fabrication process, can significantly impact device performance and yield. Developing reliable and cost-effective manufacturing processes for nanoscale components is a major hurdle for the widespread adoption of nanoelectronics [58]. Quantum computing faces even more formidable challenges in terms of scalability. Building a quantum computer with a large number of qubits that can perform meaningful calculations is a complex task. Qubits are highly sensitive to their environment, and maintaining their quantum states (coherence) over time is difficult due to noise and interference from external sources. This leads to errors in quantum computations, necessitating the development of error correction techniques, which require additional qubits and further complicate the design of quantum processors. Scaling up quantum computers to the point where they can outperform classical computers in practical applications (known as "quantum supremacy") remains an ongoing challenge [59].

The fabrication of qubits and quantum gates with high precision and uniformity across large arrays is a significant technical challenge. Quantum devices often require specialized materials and ultra-low temperatures, adding to the complexity and cost of manufacturing. Researchers are exploring various qubit technologies, such as superconducting qubits, trapped ions, and topological qubits, each with its own set of challenges related to scalability and stability. Overcoming these barriers will be critical for the transition from experimental quantum devices to practical, large-scale quantum computers. As electronic devices become smaller and more powerful, managing heat dissipation and power consumption becomes increasingly critical. In nanoelectronics, the dense packing of transistors and the high-speed operation of nanoscale devices generate significant heat, which can lead to overheating and device failure. Traditional cooling methods, such as fans and heat sinks, are becoming less effective at the nanoscale, necessitating the development of new thermal management solutions [60]. As transistors shrink, leakage currents (unintended flows of electricity) increase, leading to higher power consumption and reduced energy efficiency. To address these issues, researchers are exploring new materials and device architectures that can reduce power consumption and improve heat dissipation. For example, the use of nanomaterials like graphene and carbon nanotubes, which have high thermal conductivity, could help dissipate heat more effectively in nanoelectronic devices. Furthermore, energy-efficient computing paradigms, such as reversible computing and spintronics, are being investigated as alternatives to traditional silicon-based electronics. Quantum computing also faces challenges related to power consumption and thermal management, albeit in a different context. Quantum processors often require extremely low temperatures, close to absolute zero, to maintain the delicate quantum states of qubits. This necessitates the use of complex and energy-intensive cryogenic cooling systems, which limit the scalability and practicality of quantum computers [61]. The need for precise control and error correction in quantum operations can lead to significant power consumption, particularly as the number of qubits increases. Balancing the power requirements of quantum processors with the need for stable and low-temperature environments is a key challenge in the development of practical quantum computers. The rise of quantum computing also brings ethical and security concerns that need to be addressed as the technology matures. One of the most pressing issues is the potential for quantum computers to break current cryptographic systems, which rely on the difficulty of factoring large numbers or solving complex mathematical problems. Quantum algorithms, such as Shor's algorithm, can solve these problems exponentially faster than classical algorithms, rendering many of today's encryption methods vulnerable. This has significant implications for data security, privacy, and the integrity of digital communications. Governments, businesses, and individuals rely on encryption to protect sensitive information, and the advent of quantum computing could compromise these protections, leading to widespread cybersecurity challenges. In response to this threat, researchers are developing quantum-resistant cryptographic algorithms, known as post-quantum cryptography, to secure data against future quantum attacks [62]. However, transitioning to these new cryptographic standards will require significant time and resources, and there is a risk that quantum computers could be used maliciously before these defenses are fully in place.

FUTURE DIRECTIONS

Nanoelectronics is poised to continue evolving, driven by both the demand for higher performance and the need for energy efficiency in electronic devices. One emerging trend is the development of two-dimensional (2D) materials, such as graphene and transition metal dichalcogenides (TMDs), which offer unique electrical, thermal, and mechanical properties. These materials enable the creation of ultra-thin, flexible electronic devices that can be integrated into a variety of applications, from wearable electronics to flexible displays [63]. As researchers continue to explore the potential of 2D materials, they could play a crucial role in extending Moore's Law, allowing for further miniaturization of electronic components. Another significant trend is the rise of neuromorphic computing, which mimics the architecture of the human brain to achieve more efficient processing of complex tasks such as pattern recognition and machine learning. Nanoelectronics is essential for building neuromorphic chips, which rely on nanoscale components to replicate the behavior of neurons and synapses. These chips have the potential to revolutionize artificial intelligence (AI) by providing faster and more energy-efficient computing solutions, enabling more advanced AI systems in everything from autonomous vehicles to healthcare diagnostics [64]. In addition, spintronics, a technology that exploits the spin of electrons rather than their charge, is gaining momentum in the field of nanoelectronics. Spintronic devices, such as magnetic tunnel junctions and spin transistors, offer the promise of non-volatile memory with faster switching speeds and lower power consumption than traditional electronic devices. This could lead to the development of next-generation memory technologies that significantly improve the performance of computers and other electronic devices. The role of nanoelectronics with emerging technologies like the Internet of Things (IoT) and edge computing is another key trend. As billions of IoT devices are deployed worldwide, the demand for low-power, high-performance nanoelectronic components will grow [65]. Nanoelectronics will play a critical role in enabling smart devices and sensors that can operate efficiently at the edge of networks, processing data locally and reducing the need for centralized cloud computing.

Quantum computing is rapidly progressing from theoretical research to practical applications, with significant advancements in both hardware and software. One of the key future directions for quantum computing is the development of fault-tolerant quantum computers. Current quantum computers are prone to errors due to decoherence and noise, which limit their ability to perform complex calculations. The future of quantum computing lies in the creation of error-corrected quantum systems that can reliably perform computations at scale. Researchers are exploring various error correction codes and fault-tolerant architectures to achieve this goal, with the ultimate aim of building large-scale quantum computers that can outperform classical computers in a wide range of tasks [66]. Another important trend in quantum computing is the exploration of new qubit technologies. While superconducting qubits and trapped ions are currently the most mature platforms, other qubit technologies, such as topological qubits and photonic qubits, are being investigated for their potential to offer greater stability and scalability. Topological qubits, for example, are predicted to be more robust against errors, making them a promising candidate for building large-scale quantum computers. Photonic qubits, on the other hand, have the advantage of operating at room temperature and being compatible with existing optical communication networks, which could enable the development of quantum networks and the integration of quantum computing with classical communication systems. Quantum computing is also expected to have a profound impact on fields such as cryptography, optimization, and materials science. In cryptography, the development of quantum-resistant encryption methods will be crucial to secure communications in a post-quantum world. In optimization, quantum algorithms could revolutionize industries such as logistics, finance, and energy by providing faster and more efficient solutions to complex problems. In materials science, quantum computers could simulate the behavior of molecules and materials at the quantum level, leading to the discovery of new materials with unprecedented properties. As quantum computing continues to advance, collaboration between academia, industry, and government will be essential to overcome the technical challenges and realize the full potential of this transformative technology [67]. The development of quantum software platforms, quantum programming languages, and quantum cloud services will also play a crucial role in making quantum computing accessible to a broader range of users and applications.

The convergence of nanoelectronics and quantum computing is expected to have far-reaching implications for industry and society. In the industrial sector, nanoelectronics will continue to drive innovation in consumer electronics, telecommunications, and automotive industries. As devices become more powerful, efficient, and compact, new opportunities will arise for the development of smart products and services. The automotive industry is already exploring the use of nanoelectronics in electric vehicles (EVs) and autonomous driving systems, enabling more efficient energy management and enhanced safety features [68]. In telecommunications, nanoelectronics will be key to advancing 5G networks and beyond, enabling faster data transmission and more reliable connectivity for a growing number of devices [69]. Quantum computing, on the other hand, is poised to disrupt industries ranging from finance to healthcare. In finance, quantum computers could be used to optimize trading strategies, manage risk, and develop new financial products. In healthcare, quantum computing could accelerate drug discovery, enable personalized medicine, and improve the accuracy of medical imaging and diagnostics [70]. The ability to simulate complex biological systems at the quantum level could lead to breakthroughs in understanding diseases and developing more effective treatments. The societal implications of these technologies also raise important ethical and policy considerations. The widespread adoption of nanoelectronics and quantum computing could exacerbate existing inequalities, as access to these advanced technologies may be concentrated in the hands of a few powerful companies and nations. Ensuring that the benefits of these technologies are distributed equitably will be a key challenge for policymakers and industry leaders. The impact of quantum computing on cybersecurity and data privacy cannot be overstated. As quantum computers become capable of breaking current encryption methods, new approaches to securing sensitive information will be required. This will necessitate a global effort to develop and implement quantum-resistant cryptographic standards, as well as to educate the public and businesses about the risks and opportunities associated with quantum computing.

CONCLUSION

Nanoelectronics and quantum computing represent the cutting edge of technological innovation, offering unprecedented opportunities to enhance the performance, efficiency, and capabilities of electronic devices. Nanoelectronics has already transformed industries by enabling the miniaturization of components and the development of novel materials with unique properties. As the field continues to evolve, emerging trends such as two-dimensional materials, neuromorphic computing, and spintronics are poised to push the boundaries of what is possible, leading to smarter, more energy-efficient devices that can seamlessly integrate with other technologies like the Internet of Things. Quantum computing, on the other hand, holds the potential to revolutionize problem-solving across numerous domains, from cryptography to drug discovery. Although still in its early stages, advancements in qubit technologies, error correction, and quantum algorithms are paving the way for practical quantum computers that could solve problems far beyond the reach of classical computing. The implications for industries are profound, with quantum computing poised to disrupt finance, healthcare, logistics, and more. These advancements come with significant challenges. Manufacturing nanoelectronics at scale remains difficult, and heat dissipation and power consumption issues must be addressed to ensure the longevity of devices. Similarly, the ethical and security concerns surrounding quantum computing, particularly its impact on encryption and data privacy, require careful consideration. Looking ahead, collaboration between academia, industry, and policymakers will be crucial in navigating the challenges and realizing the full potential of these technologies. The future of nanoelectronics and quantum computing promises to reshape industries, improve lives, and solve some of the world's most pressing problems. However, it will also demand a balanced approach that prioritizes ethical considerations and equitable access to ensure that the benefits of these innovations are widely shared.

REFERENCES

[1] Baker, N.A.; Sept, D.; Joseph, S.; Holst, M.J.; McCammon, J.A. Electrostatics of nanosystems: Application to microtubules and the ribosome. *Proc. Natl. Acad. Sci. USA,* **2001**, *98*(18), 10037-10041.
[http://dx.doi.org/10.1073/pnas.181342398] [PMID: 11517324]

[2] Clauer, A.H. Laser Shock Peening, the Path to Production. *Metals (Basel),* **2019**, *9*(6), 626.
[http://dx.doi.org/10.3390/met9060626]

[3] Mudd, G.W.; Svatek, S.A.; Ren, T.; Patanè, A.; Makarovsky, O.; Eaves, L.; Beton, P.H.; Kovalyuk, Z.D.; Lashkarev, G.V.; Kudrynskyi, Z.R.; Dmitriev, A.I. Tuning the bandgap of exfoliated InSe nanosheets by quantum confinement. *Adv. Mater.,* **2013**, *25*(40), 5714-5718.
[http://dx.doi.org/10.1002/adma.201302616] [PMID: 23966225]

[4] Nanoelectronics, E. Emerging Nanoelectronics: Life with and after CMOS. *Mater. Today,* **2005**, *8*(3), 60.
[http://dx.doi.org/10.1016/S1369-7021(05)00754-6]

[5] Bogani, L. Quantum Nanoelectronics—An Introduction to Electronic Nanotechnology and Quantum Computing. By E. L. Wolf. *ChemPhysChem,* **2010**, *11*(6), 1316-1317.
[http://dx.doi.org/10.1002/cphc.200900864]

[6] Lent, C.S.; Tougaw, P.D.; Porod, W.; Bernstein, G.H. Quantum cellular automata. *Nanotechnology,* **1993**, *4*(1), 49-57.
[http://dx.doi.org/10.1088/0957-4484/4/1/004] [PMID: 21727566]

[7] Quantum mechanical effects in the design of nano-meter scale mosfets. *International Research Journal of Modernization in Engineering Technology and Science,* **2023**.
[http://dx.doi.org/10.56726/IRJMETS37718]

[8] Zhang, G.; Cheng, Y.; Ren, T.L. Multi-physics coupling in nanoscale spintronics and quantum devices. *Nanotechnology,* **2023**, *34*(50), 500202.
[http://dx.doi.org/10.1088/1361-6528/acefd6] [PMID: 37579744]

[9] Leghtas, Z.; Touzard, S.; Pop, I.M.; Kou, A.; Vlastakis, B.; Petrenko, A.; Sliwa, K.M.; Narla, A.; Shankar, S.; Hatridge, M.J.; Reagor, M.; Frunzio, L.; Schoelkopf, R.J.; Mirrahimi, M.; Devoret, M.H. Confining the state of light to a quantum manifold by engineered two-photon loss. *Science,* **2015**, *347*(6224), 853-857.
[http://dx.doi.org/10.1126/science.aaa2085] [PMID: 25700514]

[10] Anderson, B.P.; Kasevich, M.A. Macroscopic quantum interference from atomic tunnel arrays. *Science,* **1998**, *282*(5394), 1686-1689.
[http://dx.doi.org/10.1126/science.282.5394.1686] [PMID: 9831555]

[11] Valiev, M.; Bylaska, E.J.; Govind, N.; Kowalski, K.; Straatsma, T.P.; Van Dam, H.J.J.; Wang, D.; Nieplocha, J.; Apra, E.; Windus, T.L.; de Jong, W.A. NWChem: A comprehensive and scalable open-source solution for large scale molecular simulations. *Comput. Phys. Commun.,* **2010**, *181*(9), 1477-1489.
[http://dx.doi.org/10.1016/j.cpc.2010.04.018]

[12] Gisin, N.; Ribordy, G.; Tittel, W.; Zbinden, H. Quantum cryptography. *Rev. Mod. Phys.,* **2002**, *74*(1), 145-195.
[http://dx.doi.org/10.1103/RevModPhys.74.145]

[13] Lee, Y.; Kim, J.; Joo, H.; Raj, M.S.; Ghaffari, R.; Kim, D.H. Wearable sensing systems with mechanically soft assemblies of nanoscale materials. *Adv. Mater. Technol.,* **2017**, *2*(9), 1700053-1700053.
[http://dx.doi.org/10.1002/admt.201700053]

[14] V, M. Optimization of location of photoelectric modules on structures of energy efficient buildings. *Modern Problems of Modeling,* **2022**, *23*, 143-150.

[http://dx.doi.org/10.33842/2313-125X-2023-23-143-150]

[15]   O'Brien, J.L.; Furusawa, A.; Vučković, J. Photonic quantum technologies. *Nat. Photonics,* **2009**, *3*(12), 687-695.
[http://dx.doi.org/10.1038/nphoton.2009.229]

[16]   Chaudhary, A.; Chen, D.Z.; Hu, X.S.; Niemier, M.T.; Ravichandran, R.; Whitton, K. Fabricatable interconnect and molecular QCA circuits. *IEEE Trans. Comput. Aided Des. Integrated Circ. Syst.,* **2007**, *26*(11), 1978-1991.
[http://dx.doi.org/10.1109/TCAD.2007.906467]

[17]   Liebschner, D.; Afonine, P.V.; Baker, M.L.; Bunkóczi, G.; Chen, V.B.; Croll, T.I.; Hintze, B.; Hung, L.W.; Jain, S.; McCoy, A.J.; Moriarty, N.W.; Oeffner, R.D.; Poon, B.K.; Prisant, M.G.; Read, R.J.; Richardson, J.S.; Richardson, D.C.; Sammito, M.D.; Sobolev, O.V.; Stockwell, D.H.; Terwilliger, T.C.; Urzhumtsev, A.G.; Videau, L.L.; Williams, C.J.; Adams, P.D. Macromolecular structure determination using X-rays, neutrons and electrons: recent developments in *Phenix. Acta Crystallogr. D Struct. Biol.,* **2019**, *75*(10), 861-877.
[http://dx.doi.org/10.1107/S2059798319011471] [PMID: 31588918]

[18]   Acín, A.; Bloch, I.; Buhrman, H.; Calarco, T.; Eichler, C.; Eisert, J.; Esteve, D.; Gisin, N.; Glaser, S.J.; Jelezko, F.; Kuhr, S.; Lewenstein, M.; Riedel, M.F.; Schmidt, P.O.; Thew, R.; Wallraff, A.; Walmsley, I.; Wilhelm, F.K. The quantum technologies roadmap: a European community view. *New J. Phys.,* **2018**, *20*(8), 080201.
[http://dx.doi.org/10.1088/1367-2630/aad1ea]

[19]   Bennett, C.H.; DiVincenzo, D.P. Quantum information and computation. *Nature,* **2000**, *404*(6775), 247-255.
[http://dx.doi.org/10.1038/35005001] [PMID: 10749200]

[20]   Nelco, I.T.A.M.P.F.P.S. Nelco introduces two advanced materials providing faster processing speeds. *Circuit World,* **1999**, *25*(4).
[http://dx.doi.org/10.1108/cw.1999.21725dad.013]

[21]   Huang, W.; Yang, C.H.; Chan, K.W.; Tanttu, T.; Hensen, B.; Leon, R.C.C.; Fogarty, M.A.; Hwang, J.C.C.; Hudson, F.E.; Itoh, K.M.; Morello, A.; Laucht, A.; Dzurak, A.S. Fidelity benchmarks for two-qubit gates in silicon. *Nature,* **2019**, *569*(7757), 532-536.
[http://dx.doi.org/10.1038/s41586-019-1197-0] [PMID: 31086337]

[22]   Khitun, A.; Bao, M.; Wang, K.L. Magnonic logic circuits. *J. Phys. D Appl. Phys.,* **2010**, *43*(26), 264005-264005.
[http://dx.doi.org/10.1088/0022-3727/43/26/264005]

[23]   Kreutz, D.; Ramos, F.M.V.; Esteves Verissimo, P.; Esteve Rothenberg, C.; Azodolmolky, S.; Uhlig, S. Software-Defined Networking: A Comprehensive Survey. *Proc. IEEE,* **2015**, *103*(1), 14-76.
[http://dx.doi.org/10.1109/JPROC.2014.2371999]

[24]   Sharma, S.; Alam, M.A.; Sharma, A.; Singh, P.; Dhoundiyal, S.; Sharma, A. High-impact applications of iot system-based metaheuristics. In: *Nature-Inspired Methods for Smart Healthcare Systems and Medical Data*; Springer Nature: Switzerland, **2023**; pp. 121-131.

[25]   Dhoundiyal, S.; Alam, M.A.; Sagar, S.; Yadav, S.; Shadab, S.; Ahmad, N. , 10 Molecular simulations strategies for designing 2D nanomaterials for drug delivery applications. *Computational Drug Delivery: Molecular Simulation for Pharmaceutical Formulation,* **2024**; *7:* 221.

[26]   Bykovsky, A.Y.; Kompanets, I.N. Quantum cryptography and combined schemes of quantum cryptography communication networks. *Quantum Electron.,* **2018**, *48*(9), 777-801.
[http://dx.doi.org/10.1070/QEL16732]

[27]   Duncan, T.V. Applications of nanotechnology in food packaging and food safety: Barrier materials, antimicrobials and sensors. *J. Colloid Interface Sci.,* **2011**, *363*(1), 1-24.
[http://dx.doi.org/10.1016/j.jcis.2011.07.017] [PMID: 21824625]

[28]   Kretschmer, W. The Quantum Supremacy Tsirelson Inequality. *Quantum,* **2021**, *5*, 560.
       [http://dx.doi.org/10.22331/q-2021-10-07-560]

[29]   Ten Holter, C.; Inglesant, P.; Srivastava, R.; Jirotka, M. Bridging the quantum divides: a chance to
       repair classic(al) mistakes? *Quantum Sci. Technol.,* **2022**, *7*(4), 044006-044006.
       [http://dx.doi.org/10.1088/2058-9565/ac8db6]

[30]   Kong, J.; Franklin, N.R.; Zhou, C.; Chapline, M.G.; Peng, S.; Cho, K.; Dai, H. Nanotube molecular
       wires as chemical sensors. *Science,* **2000**, *287*(5453), 622-625.
       [http://dx.doi.org/10.1126/science.287.5453.622] [PMID: 10649989]

[31]   Wang, Q.H.; Kalantar-Zadeh, K.; Kis, A.; Coleman, J.N.; Strano, M.S. Electronics and optoelectronics
       of two-dimensional transition metal dichalcogenides. *Nat. Nanotechnol.,* **2012**, *7*(11), 699-712.
       [http://dx.doi.org/10.1038/nnano.2012.193] [PMID: 23132225]

[32]   Gu, H.Y.; Kim, S. Design Optimization of Double-Gate Isosceles Trapezoid Tunnel Field-Effect
       Transistor (DGIT-TFET). *Micromachines (Basel),* **2019**, *10*(4), 229.
       [http://dx.doi.org/10.3390/mi10040229] [PMID: 30935007]

[33]   Kang, K.; Min, B.I. Effect of quantum confinement on electron tunneling through a quantum dot.
       Phys. Rev. B Condens. Matter, **1997**, *55*(23), 15412-15415.
       [http://dx.doi.org/10.1103/PhysRevB.55.15412]

[34]   Cha, C.; Shin, S.R.; Annabi, N.; Dokmeci, M.R.; Khademhosseini, A. Carbon-based nanomaterials:
       multifunctional materials for biomedical engineering. *ACS Nano,* **2013**, *7*(4), 2891-2897.
       [http://dx.doi.org/10.1021/nn401196a] [PMID: 23560817]

[35]   Klaine, S.J.; Koelmans, A.A.; Horne, N.; Carley, S.; Handy, R.D.; Kapustka, L.; Nowack, B.; von der
       Kammer, F. Paradigms to assess the environmental impact of manufactured nanomaterials. *Environ.
       Toxicol. Chem.,* **2012**, *31*(1), 3-14.
       [http://dx.doi.org/10.1002/etc.733] [PMID: 22162122]

[36]   Mushtaq, U.; Akram, M. W.; Prasad, D. FinFET: A revolution in nanometer regime. *Lecture Notes in
       Electrical Engineering,* **2022**, 403-417.
       [http://dx.doi.org/10.1007/978-981-19-4300-3_35]

[37]   Colinge, J.P.; Lee, C.W.; Afzalian, A.; Akhavan, N.D.; Yan, R.; Ferain, I.; Razavi, P.; O'Neill, B.;
       Blake, A.; White, M.; Kelleher, A.M.; McCarthy, B.; Murphy, R. Nanowire transistors without
       junctions. *Nat. Nanotechnol.,* **2010**, *5*(3), 225-229.
       [http://dx.doi.org/10.1038/nnano.2010.15] [PMID: 20173755]

[38]   Zwanenburg, F.A.; Dzurak, A.S.; Morello, A.; Simmons, M.Y.; Hollenberg, L.C.L.; Klimeck, G.;
       Rogge, S.; Coppersmith, S.N.; Eriksson, M.A. Silicon quantum electronics. *Rev. Mod. Phys.,* **2013**,
       85(3), 961-1019.
       [http://dx.doi.org/10.1103/RevModPhys.85.961]

[39]   Hsu, C.W.; Zhen, B.; Stone, A.D.; Joannopoulos, J.D.; Soljačić, M. Bound states in the continuum.
       Nat. Rev. Mater., **2016**, *1*(9), 16048.
       [http://dx.doi.org/10.1038/natrevmats.2016.48]

[40]   Takahashi, Y.; Fujiwara, A.; Yamazaki, K.; Namatsu, H.; Kurihara, K.; Murase, K. A Si Memory
       Device Composed of a One-Dimensional Metal-Oxide-Semiconductor Field-Effect-Transistor Switch
       and a Single-Electron-Transistor Detector. *Jpn. J. Appl. Phys.,* **1999**, *38*(4S), 2457-2457.
       [http://dx.doi.org/10.1143/JJAP.38.2457]

[41]   Wang, J.; Meng, H.; Wang, J.P. Programmable spintronics logic device based on a magnetic tunnel
       junction element. *J. Appl. Phys.,* **2005**, *97*(10), 10D509.
       [http://dx.doi.org/10.1063/1.1857655]

[42]   Freeman, R.; Willner, I. Optical molecular sensing with semiconductor quantum dots (QDs). *Chem.
       Soc. Rev.,* **2012**, *41*(10), 4067-4085.
       [http://dx.doi.org/10.1039/c2cs15357b] [PMID: 22481608]

[43]   Yen, B.K.H.; Günther, A.; Schmidt, M.A.; Jensen, K.F.; Bawendi, M.G. A microfabricated gas-liquid segmented flow reactor for high-temperature synthesis: The case of CdSe quantum dots. *Angew. Chem. Int. Ed.,* **2005**, *44*(34), 5447-5451.
[http://dx.doi.org/10.1002/anie.200500792]

[44]   Darr, J.A.; Zhang, J.; Makwana, N.M.; Weng, X. Continuous hydrothermal synthesis of inorganic nanoparticles: applications and future directions. *Chem. Rev.,* **2017**, *117*(17), 11125-11238.
[http://dx.doi.org/10.1021/acs.chemrev.6b00417] [PMID: 28771006]

[45]   Reina, A.; Jia, X.; Ho, J.; Nezich, D.; Son, H.; Bulovic, V.; Dresselhaus, M.S.; Kong, J. Large area, few-layer graphene films on arbitrary substrates by chemical vapor deposition. *Nano Lett.,* **2009**, *9*(1), 30-35.
[http://dx.doi.org/10.1021/nl801827v] [PMID: 19046078]

[46]   Sharma, P.; Mehta, M.; Dhanjal, D.S.; Kaur, S.; Gupta, G.; Singh, H.; Thangavelu, L.; Rajeshkumar, S.; Tambuwala, M.; Bakshi, H.A.; Chellappan, D.K.; Dua, K.; Satija, S. Emerging trends in the novel drug delivery approaches for the treatment of lung cancer. *Chem. Biol. Interact.,* **2019**, *309*, 108720.
[http://dx.doi.org/10.1016/j.cbi.2019.06.033] [PMID: 31226287]

[47]   Groenendaal, L.; Jonas, F.; Freitag, D.; Pielartzik, H.; Reynolds, J.R. Poly(3,4-ethylenedioxythiophene) and Its Derivatives: Past, Present, and Future. *Adv. Mater.,* **2000**, *12*(7), 481-494.
[http://dx.doi.org/10.1002/(SICI)1521-4095(200004)12:7<481::AID-ADMA481>3.0.CO;2-C]

[48]   Loss, D.; DiVincenzo, D.P. Quantum computation with quantum dots. *Phys. Rev. A,* **1998**, *57*(1), 120-126.
[http://dx.doi.org/10.1103/PhysRevA.57.120]

[49]   Ceña, V.; Játiva, P. Nanoparticle crossing of blood-brain barrier: a road to new therapeutic approaches to central nervous system diseases. *Nanomedicine (Lond.),* **2018**, *13*(13), 1513-1516.
[http://dx.doi.org/10.2217/nnm-2018-0139] [PMID: 29998779]

[50]   Grover, L.K. A fast quantum mechanical algorithm for database search. **1996**.
[http://dx.doi.org/10.1145/237814.237866]

[51]   Gurnyak, I. Using cloud services google forms and microsoft forms in the teaching process. *Physical and Mathematical Education,* **2018**, *16*(2), 40-45.
[http://dx.doi.org/10.31110/2413-1571-2018-016-2-008]

[52]   Aaronson, S.; Gottesman, D. Improved simulation of stabilizer circuits. *Phys. Rev. A,* **2004**, *70*(5), 052328.
[http://dx.doi.org/10.1103/PhysRevA.70.052328]

[53]   Barad, K. Quantum entanglements and hauntological relations of inheritance: Dis/continuities, spacetime enfoldings, and justice-to-come. *Derrida Today,* **2010**, *3*(2), 240-268.
[http://dx.doi.org/10.3366/drt.2010.0206]

[54]   Dorota Rymaszewska, A. The challenges of lean manufacturing implementation in SMEs. *Benchmarking (Bradf.),* **2014**, *21*(6), 987-1002.
[http://dx.doi.org/10.1108/BIJ-10-2012-0065]

[55]   Gisin, N.; Ribordy, G.; Tittel, W.; Zbinden, H. Quantum cryptography. *Rev. Mod. Phys.,* **2002**, *74*(1), 145-195.
[http://dx.doi.org/10.1103/RevModPhys.74.145]

[56]   Khan, H.N.; Hounshell, D.A.; Fuchs, E.R.H. Science and research policy at the end of Moore's law. *Nat. Electron.,* **2018**, *1*(1), 14-21.
[http://dx.doi.org/10.1038/s41928-017-0005-9]

[57]   Hassija, V.; Chamola, V.; Saxena, V.; Chanana, V.; Parashari, P.; Mumtaz, S.; Guizani, M. Present landscape of quantum computing. *IET Quantum Commun.,* **2020**, *1*(2), 42-48.
[http://dx.doi.org/10.1049/iet-qtc.2020.0027]

[58]   Kolb, H.C.; Finn, M.G.; Sharpless, K.B. Click Chemistry: Diverse Chemical Function from a Few Good Reactions. *Angew. Chem. Int. Ed.,* **2001**, *40*(11), 2004-2021.
[http://dx.doi.org/10.1002/1521-3773(20010601)40:11<2004::AID-ANIE2004>3.0.CO;2-5]   [PMID: 11433435]

[59]   Joshi, S.; Moazeni, S. Scaling up superconducting quantum computers with cryogenic RF-photonics. *J. Lightwave Technol.,* **2024**, *42*(1), 166-175.
[http://dx.doi.org/10.1109/JLT.2023.3311806]

[60]   Kirkpatrick, S.; Gelatt, C.D., Jr; Vecchi, M.P. Optimization by simulated annealing. *Science,* **1983**, *220*(4598), 671-680.
[http://dx.doi.org/10.1126/science.220.4598.671] [PMID: 17813860]

[61]   Hasan, M.Z.; Kane, C.L. *Colloquium* : Topological insulators. *Rev. Mod. Phys.,* **2010**, *82*(4), 3045-3067.
[http://dx.doi.org/10.1103/RevModPhys.82.3045]

[62]   Witte, K. Fear control and danger control: A test of the extended parallel process model (EPPM). *Commun. Monogr.,* **1994**, *61*(2), 113-134.
[http://dx.doi.org/10.1080/03637759409376328]

[63]   Swan, M. The quantified self: Fundamental disruption in big data science and biological discovery. *Big Data,* **2013**, *1*(2), 85-99.
[http://dx.doi.org/10.1089/big.2012.0002] [PMID: 27442063]

[64]   Chowdhury, U. K. How nanotechnology can revolutionize drug delivery. *Journal of Artificial intelligence and Machine Learning,* **2023**, *1*(1), 1-2.
[http://dx.doi.org/10.55124/jaim.v1i1.235]

[65]   Hulaj, A. Compressing big data generated by IoT devices deployed along the green borderline. *Przegląd Elektrotechniczny,* **2023**, *1*(12), 111-115.
[http://dx.doi.org/10.15199/48.2023.12.20]

[66]   Zhou, S.; Liu, Z.W.; Jiang, L. New perspectives on covariant quantum error correction. *Quantum,* **2021**, *5*, 521.
[http://dx.doi.org/10.22331/q-2021 08-09-521]

[67]   Salomon-Ferrer, R.; Case, D.A.; Walker, R.C. An overview of the Amber biomolecular simulation package. *Wiley Interdiscip. Rev. Comput. Mol. Sci.,* **2013**, *3*(2), 198-210.
[http://dx.doi.org/10.1002/wcms.1121]

[68]   Fuller, J.; Bartl, M.; Ernst, H.; Muhlbacher, H. Community based innovation: A method to utilize the innovative potential of online communities. *37th Annual Hawaii International Conference on System Sciences, 2004. Proceedings of the,* **2004**.
[http://dx.doi.org/10.1109/HICSS.2004.1265464]

[69]   Advanced wireless networks vision and future of 5g wireless mobile technology. *International Journal of Recent Trends in Engineering and Research,* **2018**, *4*(3), 141-149.
[http://dx.doi.org/10.23883/IJRTER.2018.4108.V9XYD]

[70]   Dash, S.; Shakyawar, S.K.; Sharma, M.; Kaushik, S. Big data in healthcare: management, analysis and future prospects. *J. Big Data,* **2019**, *6*(1), 54.
[http://dx.doi.org/10.1186/s40537-019-0217-0]

CHAPTER 6

Exploring Space with Nanotechnology Innovations

Abstract: Nanotechnology is revolutionizing space exploration by offering innovative solutions to some of the most challenging aspects of space travel. This paper explores the role of nanotechnology in enhancing spacecraft design, sensor technology, and mission capabilities. Lightweight nanomaterials, such as carbon nanotubes, graphene-based materials, and nano-composites, are pivotal in reducing spacecraft weight while increasing strength and durability, enabling more efficient missions. Nano-sensors and instruments, with their miniaturization, increased sensitivity, and energy efficiency, are transforming data collection and analysis in space. The application of nanotechnology extends to deep space exploration, satellite systems, and space propulsion, where it plays a critical role in long-duration missions, radiation protection, and energy harvesting. Despite its promise, challenges such as manufacturing scalability and material durability in extreme environments must be addressed. However, ongoing innovations and collaborations between space agencies and nanotechnology experts present exciting opportunities for the future. This chapter provides an in-depth examination of the current and potential impact of nanotechnology on space exploration, highlighting its significance in driving the next generation of space missions and ensuring the success of ambitious ventures beyond Earth.

Keywords: Carbon nanotubes, Cubesats, Earth, Graphene, Mars, Space exploration.

INTRODUCTION

Nanotechnology has emerged as a game-changer in the field of space exploration, offering solutions to many of the challenges that have traditionally limited humanity's reach into space. Nanotechnology in space involves the use of nanoscale materials, devices, and systems that operate at dimensions typically less than 100 nanometers. At this scale, materials often exhibit unique properties—such as increased strength, enhanced conductivity, and improved thermal resistance—that can be exploited to create more efficient and durable space technologies [1]. For example, carbon nanotubes are over 100 times stronger than steel but only a fraction of the weight, making them ideal for constructing spacecraft components that need to be both robust and lightweight. Graphene, another nanomaterial, is not only incredibly strong but also highly conductive, which makes it suitable for use in advanced electronics and thermal

Shivang Dhoundiyal & Aftab Alam

management systems within spacecraft [2]. These materials help reduce the mass of spacecraft, lowering the cost of launches, which is a critical factor in space missions. Nanotechnology also facilitates the development of nano-scale sensors and instruments that can be integrated into spacecraft to perform functions that were previously impossible or impractical. These include nanoscale chemical sensors that can detect and analyze gases in a planet's atmosphere, radiation detectors that are more sensitive than traditional devices, and nano-optical sensors that can capture high-resolution images with minimal power consumption [3]. The small size of these devices allows for their deployment in large numbers, providing redundancy and increasing the reliability of data collection in space missions. The miniaturization enabled by nanotechnology is crucial for missions involving small satellites, such as CubeSats, which are increasingly used for scientific research, Earth observation, and communication purposes [4]. The importance of nanotechnology for future missions lies in its ability to address the complex requirements of space exploration as humanity pushes further into the cosmos. As we plan for more ambitious goals, such as establishing a human presence on Mars, mining asteroids for resources, and exploring the outer planets, traditional technologies may fall short in terms of efficiency, durability, and cost-effectiveness. Nanotechnology offers solutions that can meet these demands. For instance, long-duration missions to distant planets or asteroids will require spacecraft that can survive extreme conditions, including intense radiation, micrometeoroid impacts, and temperature fluctuations. Nanomaterials can be engineered to provide enhanced radiation shielding, reducing the risk to both astronauts and equipment. Additionally, self-healing nanomaterials could repair damage from micrometeoroid impacts autonomously, extending the lifespan of spacecraft and reducing the need for maintenance. Nanotechnology also promises significant advancements in energy management and propulsion systems for future missions. Nano-coatings and nanostructured materials can improve the efficiency of solar panels, allowing spacecraft to generate more power from the same amount of sunlight [5]. This is particularly important for missions to the outer planets, where sunlight is much weaker. In propulsion, nanoscale fuels and catalysts can provide more efficient reactions, reducing the amount of fuel needed for long journeys and enabling spacecraft to travel further with less mass. Another critical area where nanotechnology can contribute is in life support systems for manned missions. Nanoscale filters and purification systems can provide more effective recycling of air and water, ensuring that astronauts have a sustainable supply of essential resources during long missions. Nano-enhanced medical devices and drug delivery systems could also improve the health and safety of astronauts by providing rapid diagnostics and targeted treatments for medical conditions that may arise in space.

LIGHTWEIGHT MATERIALS FOR SPACECRAFT

The need for lightweight materials in spacecraft design is driven by the fundamental challenges of space exploration, particularly the high costs and energy demands associated with launching and operating spacecraft. Every kilogram of payload launched into space requires a significant amount of fuel, making weight reduction a top priority for space agencies and private companies. Lightweight materials not only lower launch costs but also increase the efficiency of spacecraft, allowing for more scientific instruments, fuel, or cargo to be carried without exceeding weight limits, as highlighted by different case studies in Table 6.1. This is especially critical for long-duration missions where every gram counts in optimizing spacecraft performance. In addition to reducing launch costs, lightweight materials also contribute to the overall durability and safety of spacecraft. For example, materials like carbon nanotubes and graphene can provide exceptional strength-to-weight ratios, which means that spacecraft can withstand the harsh conditions of space, such as micrometeoroid impacts, extreme temperatures, and radiation, without adding unnecessary mass [6]. These materials can also improve fuel efficiency in propulsion systems by reducing the overall mass of the spacecraft, which allows for greater speed and maneuverability with the same amount of fuel. Lightweight materials are crucial for modular spacecraft design, where components can be easily assembled and disassembled in space. This flexibility is vital for missions that require on-orbit construction, such as building space stations or assembling spacecraft for deep-space exploration. By reducing the mass of individual components, nanomaterials make it easier to transport and assemble complex structures in space.

Table 6.1. Case Studies: Successful applications of lightweight nanomaterials in space missions.

Mission/Project	Nanomaterial Used	Application	Benefits	Outcome/Impact	References
NASA's MSL Curiosity Rover	Carbon Nanotubes	Structural components and lightweight wiring	Reduced weight, enhanced durability	Increased payload capacity and mission longevity	[7]
ESA's Sentinel Satellites	Graphene-Based Materials	Thermal control systems	Improved thermal management, reduced material bulk	Enhanced performance in harsh space environments	[8]
NASA's Solar Probe Plus	Nano-Composites	Heat shield construction	High strength-to-weight ratio, excellent insulation	Successfully withstood extreme solar temperatures	[9]

(Table 6.1) cont.....

Mission/Project	Nanomaterial Used	Application	Benefits	Outcome/Impact	References
JAXA's IKAROS Solar Sail	Nano-coatings	Lightweight solar sail membrane	Increased efficiency in solar propulsion	Demonstrated practical use of lightweight sails for deep space travel	[10]
SpaceX's Starship	Advanced Nano-alloys	Structural frames and components	Lightweight yet robust construction	Improved fuel efficiency and reduced launch costs.	[11]

Types of Nanomaterials for Spacecraft

Nanomaterials are at the forefront of innovation in spacecraft design, offering unparalleled advantages in terms of strength, weight reduction, and resilience to the harsh conditions of space. These materials enable engineers to push the boundaries of what is possible in space exploration, allowing for the creation of spacecraft that are lighter, more durable, and more efficient [12]. Below are some of the most promising types of nanomaterials currently being explored for use in spacecraft. Carbon nanotubes (CNTs) are cylindrical nanostructures composed of carbon atoms arranged in a hexagonal lattice. They are one of the strongest materials known, with a tensile strength over 100 times that of steel while being only a fraction of the weight [13]. This exceptional strength-to-weight ratio makes CNTs ideal for use in spacecraft structures, where minimizing mass without sacrificing durability is critical. In addition to their strength, CNTs exhibit excellent electrical and thermal conductivity, which can be leveraged in spacecraft wiring, sensors, and thermal management systems. CNTs are also resistant to radiation and extreme temperatures, making them suitable for space environments where materials must endure harsh conditions over extended periods. Applications of CNTs in spacecraft include the construction of lightweight structural components, electromagnetic shielding, and the reinforcement of other materials to enhance their mechanical properties.

Graphene is a single layer of carbon atoms arranged in a two-dimensional honeycomb lattice, and it is another nanomaterial that holds tremendous promise for spacecraft applications. Graphene is incredibly strong, even stronger than carbon nanotubes in some respects, and it is also highly flexible and lightweight. Its exceptional electrical conductivity makes it an ideal material for advanced electronics and energy storage systems in spacecraft. For example, graphene-based supercapacitors can store and release energy much more efficiently than traditional batteries, which is crucial for powering spacecraft systems during long missions. Additionally, graphene's thermal conductivity helps dissipate heat effectively, which is essential for managing temperature fluctuations in space

[14]. Its transparency and flexibility also open possibilities for use in flexible solar panels and lightweight, durable spacecraft windows. The combination of these properties makes graphene-based materials versatile for a wide range of applications, from structural components to electronic devices in space exploration.

Nano-composites are materials that combine nanoparticles with traditional materials to enhance their properties. These composites can be tailored to exhibit a combination of strength, flexibility, and resistance to extreme conditions, making them highly suitable for spacecraft. For instance, incorporating carbon nanotubes or graphene into polymer matrices can produce composites that are both lightweight and incredibly strong, with improved thermal and electrical properties. Nano-composites are also valuable for creating multifunctional materials, where a single material can perform multiple roles, such as providing structural support while also serving as a thermal insulator or electromagnetic shield [15]. This multifunctionality is particularly advantageous in spacecraft design, where space and weight are at a premium. Applications of nano-composites in space include protective coatings, structural components, and materials for radiation shielding.

Metal oxide nanoparticles, such as titanium dioxide (TiO_2) and zinc oxide (ZnO), are being explored for their potential in spacecraft applications, particularly in the areas of energy generation and environmental protection. TiO_2 nanoparticles are used in the development of advanced photovoltaic cells, which can convert solar energy into electricity more efficiently than traditional solar panels [16]. This is particularly important for long-duration missions where reliable energy sources are essential. Additionally, metal oxide nanoparticles have photocatalytic properties, meaning they can break down harmful organic compounds when exposed to light. This can be used to develop self-cleaning surfaces and air purification systems in spacecraft, helping to maintain a clean and safe environment for astronauts.

Boron nitride nanotubes (BNNTs) are structurally similar to carbon nanotubes but consist of boron and nitrogen atoms. BNNTs offer a unique combination of properties, including high thermal conductivity, excellent chemical stability, and the ability to withstand high temperatures [17]. Unlike carbon nanotubes, BNNTs are electrically insulating, which makes them useful for applications requiring thermal management without electrical conduction. In spacecraft, BNNTs can be used in thermal protection systems to shield components from the intense heat generated during re-entry or in the vicinity of the sun. Their chemical stability also makes them resistant to corrosion, a valuable property for spacecraft exposed to the space environment.

Fullerenes are a class of carbon-based nanomaterials that form spherical, hollow structures. They exhibit unique mechanical, electrical, and thermal properties that make them attractive for various space applications. Fullerenes can be used in the development of lightweight, strong materials that also provide protection against radiation [18]. In addition, fullerenes are being studied for their potential in drug delivery systems for space medicine, where targeted delivery of therapeutics could be crucial for astronaut health on long missions.

Fig. (**6.1**) represents the roadmap provided by the scientists at NASA on how they will be using nanotechnology in exploring celestial data.

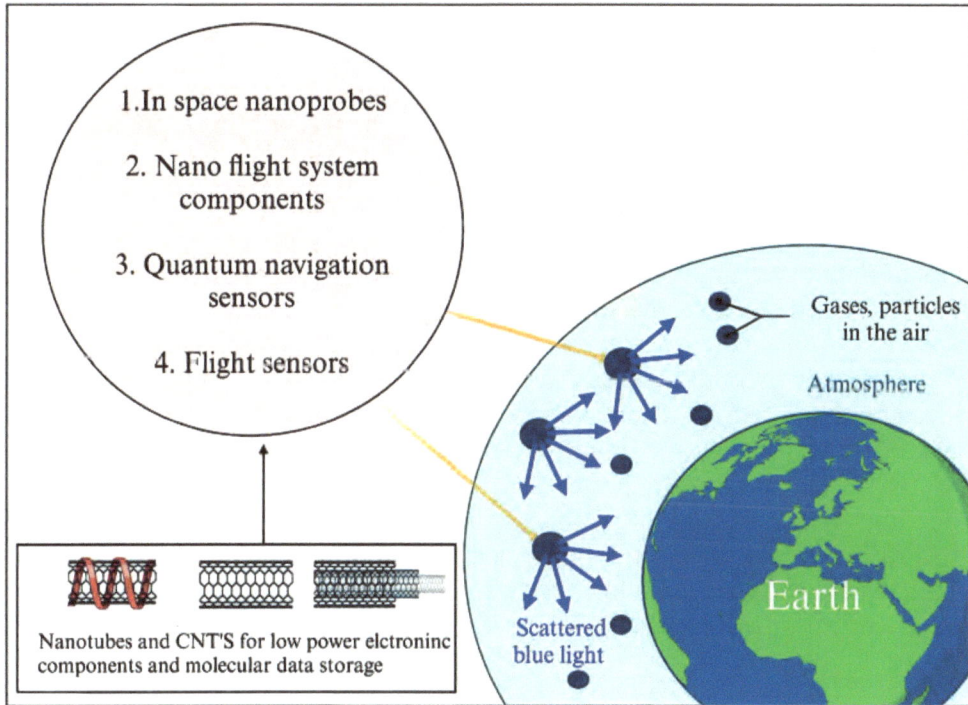

Fig. (6.1). Brief representation of NASA's nanotechnology roadmap.

Benefits of using Nanomaterials in Spacecraft

The use of nanomaterials in spacecraft design offers several transformative benefits that address critical challenges in space exploration. These benefits are primarily centered around reduced weight, enhanced strength and durability, and thermal management properties, all of which contribute to the overall efficiency, safety, and success of space missions. One of the most significant advantages of using nanomaterials in spacecraft is the substantial reduction in weight they offer [19]. Traditional spacecraft materials, such as metals and composites, are often heavy, leading to higher fuel requirements and increased launch costs. This weight reduction directly translates into lower launch costs, as less fuel is needed to propel a lighter spacecraft into orbit. Additionally, the saved weight can be allocated to carrying additional scientific instruments, cargo, or fuel, thereby extending the mission's capabilities and duration. In long-duration missions, where every gram counts, the use of lightweight nanomaterials can make a significant difference in mission success. In the unforgiving environment of space, where extreme temperatures, radiation, and micrometeoroid impacts are constant threats, the strength and durability of spacecraft materials are paramount. Nanomaterials excel in these areas, offering enhanced mechanical properties that surpass those of traditional materials [20]. These properties are particularly valuable for long-term missions, where the spacecraft must remain operational for extended periods without the possibility of maintenance or repair. The enhanced strength and durability provided by nanomaterials ensure that spacecraft can endure the harsh conditions of space, reducing the risk of mission failure due to material degradation. Effective thermal management is crucial in spacecraft design, as temperatures in space can vary widely, from the extreme cold of deep space to the intense heat generated during re-entry or exposure to direct sunlight. Nanomaterials offer superior thermal management properties that help maintain the optimal temperature of spacecraft systems and components [21]. This property is especially important for preventing overheating of sensitive electronics and instruments, which could otherwise malfunction or fail. Additionally, boron nitride nanotubes (BNNTs) are another nanomaterial with exceptional thermal conductivity, along with the added benefit of being electrically insulating. This makes BNNTs ideal for thermal protection systems, where managing heat without conducting electricity is critical. By integrating these nanomaterials into spacecraft design, engineers can better control the thermal environment, ensuring that all systems operate within their required temperature ranges, which is essential for mission success.

NANO-SENSORS AND INSTRUMENTS

Nano-sensors are a groundbreaking innovation in space exploration, offering enhanced sensitivity, miniaturization, and efficiency in detecting and measuring various environmental and physiological parameters. In the context of space missions, nano-sensors are vital for monitoring the spacecraft's internal environment, assessing external conditions, and ensuring the health and safety of astronauts, as highlighted by different examples in Table **6.2**. Due to their small size, nano-sensors can be unified into various systems and components without adding significant weight or bulk, which is a critical consideration for spacecraft design. For example, nano-sensors can detect changes in temperature, pressure, and radiation levels with extreme precision, providing real-time data that is crucial for making informed decisions during a mission [22]. This capability is especially important in deep space missions, where immediate responses to environmental changes can be life-saving. Nano-sensors are instrumental in scientific research conducted in space. They can be used to analyze the composition of extraterrestrial atmospheres, detect the presence of life-supporting molecules, and monitor cosmic radiation levels. The high sensitivity of nanosensors enables the detection of trace amounts of gases or particles, which is essential for studying distant planets and moons. In addition, nano-sensors are used in health monitoring systems for astronauts, where they can track vital signs, detect early signs of illness, or monitor the effectiveness of treatments in the microgravity environment of space. By providing continuous and accurate data, nano-sensors contribute to the success of long-term missions and the well-being of the crew.

Table 6.2. Examples of nano-instruments in current and upcoming missions.

Mission/Project	Nano-instrument	Function	Key Features	Mission Objective	References
NASA's Mars 2020 Perseverance	Nano-based Radiation Detectors	Detect and measure radiation levels on Mars	High sensitivity, low power consumption.	Assessing Mars' habitability and potential human exploration.	[23]
ESA's JUICE Mission	Nano-optical Sensors	Detect light and radiation in Jupiter's icy moons.	High precision, miniaturized size	Study the environment and potential habitability of moons	[24]
NASA's Artemis Program	Nanoscale Chemical Sensors	Monitor atmospheric conditions and detect gases	Rapid response time, ultra-compact design	Ensuring safety for crewed lunar missions	[25]
ISRO's Chandrayaan-3	Nano-spectrometers	Analyze lunar surface composition	Enhanced resolution, compact form	High-precision mapping of the lunar surface	[26]
NASA's Dragonfly Mission	Nano-gravimeters	Measure gravity variations on Titan	Lightweight, high accuracy	Exploring Titan's atmosphere and surface	[27]

Types of Nano-sensors used in Space

The role of nano-sensors in space exploration missions has significantly advanced the ability to monitor, detect, and analyze various environmental and physiological parameters in space. These sensors are designed to be highly sensitive, compact, and capable of operating under the extreme conditions of space. Below are some of the key types of nano-sensors used in space exploration, each tailored for specific applications that enhance the safety and success of missions.

Nanoscale chemical sensors are designed to detect and analyze chemical compounds with high precision and sensitivity. In space exploration, these sensors are crucial for monitoring the spacecraft's environment and detecting potentially hazardous gases or chemical leaks [28]. For example, nanoscale chemical sensors can detect trace amounts of oxygen, carbon dioxide, or other volatile organic compounds (VOCs) that might indicate a malfunction in the life support system or the presence of contaminants. These sensors utilize nanomaterials such as metal oxides, carbon nanotubes, or graphene, which exhibit excellent surface area-to-volume ratios, allowing them to interact with and detect even minute concentrations of chemicals [29]. Additionally, nanoscale chemical sensors can be deployed in planetary exploration missions to analyze the composition of extraterrestrial atmospheres or soil, helping scientists understand the chemical makeup of other planets and moons. This information is vital for assessing the habitability of these celestial bodies and for detecting signs of life.

Space is filled with various forms of radiation, including cosmic rays, solar radiation, and high-energy particles from distant stars. Nano-based radiation detectors are essential for protecting both astronauts and spacecraft from the harmful effects of this radiation [30]. Traditional radiation detectors are often bulky and consume significant power, but nano-based detectors offer a more compact and energy-efficient solution. These detectors utilize materials like nanocrystals, quantum dots, or nanocomposites, which have enhanced sensitivity to different types of radiation. For example, nanocrystal-based detectors can detect gamma rays, X-rays, and other ionizing radiation with high accuracy, allowing for real-time monitoring of radiation levels inside and outside the spacecraft. This is particularly important for long-duration missions, where cumulative radiation exposure can pose serious health risks to astronauts. Additionally, nano-based radiation detectors can be used to study cosmic radiation, providing valuable data for understanding the radiation environment in space and developing better protective measures for future missions [31].

Nano-optical sensors play a critical role in space exploration by enabling precise measurements of light, imaging, and detection of optical phenomena. These sensors are built using nanomaterials like plasmonic nanoparticles, photonic crystals, or nanowires, which enhance their ability to interact with light at the nanoscale. In space missions, nano-optical sensors are used for a variety of applications, including navigation, communication, and scientific research. For example, these sensors can detect changes in light intensity, polarization, or wavelength, providing crucial information for tasks such as aligning spacecraft, tracking celestial bodies, or monitoring the Sun's activity [32]. Nano-optical sensors are also used in telescopes and imaging systems to capture high-resolution images of distant stars, galaxies, and other celestial objects. Their small size allows them to be integrated into compact, lightweight instruments, making them ideal for use in space probes, satellites, and landers. Additionally, nano-optical sensors can be employed in experiments that study the properties of light in the vacuum of space, contributing to our understanding of fundamental physics.

In addition to the chemical, radiation, and optical sensors, several other types of nanosensors are used in space exploration to address specific challenges. Nano-electromechanical systems (NEMS), for example, are miniature devices that combine mechanical and electrical components at the nanoscale [33]. These systems can be used for precise motion sensing, vibration detection, or force measurements, which are critical for tasks such as spacecraft docking, deploying instruments, or analyzing mechanical properties of materials. NEMS devices are known for their high sensitivity and low power consumption, making them ideal for long-duration missions where energy efficiency is paramount.

Nano-biosensors are another important category, particularly in missions involving human astronauts. These sensors can monitor biological parameters, such as glucose levels, heart rate, or stress markers, ensuring that astronauts remain in good health during their journey [34]. Nano-biosensors can also detect pathogens or contaminants in the spacecraft environment, helping to prevent the spread of infections in the confined space of a spacecraft. Magnetic nanosensors are utilized for detecting magnetic fields and their variations. These sensors are valuable in space missions for tasks like studying planetary magnetospheres, detecting magnetic anomalies on the Moon or Mars, and navigating spacecraft through magnetic fields [35].

Advantages of Nano-sensors in Space Exploration

Nano-sensors offer several key advantages in space exploration, significantly enhancing mission efficiency, safety, and scientific capabilities. Each of these benefits plays a crucial role in addressing the challenges of space missions, where every aspect of design and performance is critical to success. One of the most significant advantages of nano-sensors in space exploration is their ability to be miniaturized without compromising performance [36]. Traditional sensors and instruments often occupy considerable space and add substantial weight to spacecraft, which is a major concern given the cost and energy requirements of launching heavy payloads. Nano-sensors, on the other hand, can be produced at a fraction of the size and weight of conventional sensors due to their nanoscale dimensions and the use of nanomaterials like carbon nanotubes, quantum dots, and nanowires. This miniaturization allows for more sensors to be packed into a spacecraft, enabling comprehensive monitoring and data collection while still adhering to strict weight limitations [37]. Additionally, the reduction in sensor size allows for more compact and streamlined designs, which can improve the overall aerodynamics and fuel efficiency of spacecraft. Miniaturization is particularly valuable for small satellites (CubeSats) and probes, where space is limited, and every gram of weight saved is critical for mission success [38]. Nano-sensors offer vastly superior sensitivity and precision compared to their traditional counterparts, making them invaluable for detecting minute changes in the space environment. The unique properties of nanomaterials, such as high surface area-to-volume ratios and quantum effects, enable these sensors to detect extremely low concentrations of gases, chemicals, or radiation that would be undetectable by conventional sensors. For example, nano-chemical sensors can identify trace amounts of volatile organic compounds or toxic gases within a spacecraft, providing early warnings that can prevent life-threatening situations [39]. Similarly, nano-based radiation detectors can precisely measure subtle variations in radiation levels, offering critical data for both crew safety and scientific research. This heightened sensitivity and precision also extend to nano-optical sensors, which can capture detailed images and detect changes in light intensity with unparalleled accuracy. By providing more accurate and reliable data, nano-sensors enhance the ability to monitor and respond to the dynamic conditions of space, leading to better-informed decisions and more successful missions. Energy efficiency is a paramount consideration in space exploration, where power resources are limited, and every watt of energy must be used judiciously [40]. Nano-sensors excel in this area due to their low power consumption, which stems from their small size and the efficiency of the nanomaterials used in their construction. Unlike traditional sensors that may require significant power to operate, nano-sensors can function with minimal energy, often relying on the inherent properties of nanomaterials that enable passive sensing or require only small amounts of electrical input. This energy efficiency is particularly beneficial for long-duration missions, where conserving power is critical to extending the operational life of the spacecraft and its instruments [41]. Additionally, the reduced energy demands of nano-sensors allow for the allocation of more power to other mission-critical systems, such as communication, propulsion, and life support. In solar-powered spacecraft, where energy availability fluctuates based on distance from the Sun, the energy efficiency of nano-sensors ensures continuous operation even in low-power conditions [42]. This efficiency supports the development of autonomous or semi-autonomous systems that can operate for extended periods without direct human intervention, making nano-sensors ideal for deep-space exploration and planetary missions.

ENHANCING SPACE MISSIONS WITH NANOTECHNOLOGY

As humanity ventures beyond Earth's orbit and embarks on deep space missions, nanotechnology plays a pivotal role in overcoming the unique challenges associated with long-duration space exploration [43]. The harsh environment of deep space, including exposure to high levels of cosmic radiation, extreme temperatures, and the prolonged isolation of astronauts, demands innovative solutions that can enhance the safety, sustainability, and success of these missions. Nanotechnology offers advanced materials and systems that address these critical needs, making it an indispensable tool for the future of deep space exploration.

Long-duration space missions, such as those to Mars, asteroids, or beyond, require spacecraft and systems that can endure the rigors of space for extended periods, often lasting months or years [44]. Nanotechnology contributes to the development of lightweight, durable materials that reduce the overall mass of spacecraft, thereby lowering fuel consumption and extending mission duration. For instance, nanomaterials like carbon nanotubes and graphene composites are used to construct spacecraft components that are both stronger and lighter than traditional materials, improving the structural integrity of the spacecraft while reducing weight. Additionally, nanotechnology enables the creation of self-healing materials that can automatically repair small cracks or damage caused by micrometeoroids or space debris, ensuring the spacecraft remains operational over long missions. Nanotechnology also plays a critical role in life support systems for astronauts on long-duration missions. Nano-based filtration systems can purify air and water with high efficiency, removing contaminants and recycling resources to sustain the crew [45]. In addition, nano-sensors can monitor the spacecraft's environment in real-time, detecting changes in temperature, humidity, and atmospheric composition, and alerting the crew to any potential issues. These innovations are essential for maintaining a habitable environment within the spacecraft for the duration of the mission, reducing the risk of system failures that could jeopardize the crew's safety.

Radiation exposure is one of the most significant threats to the health of astronauts on deep space missions. Unlike Earth, which is protected by its magnetic field and atmosphere, deep space offers no natural protection from cosmic rays, solar radiation, and other high-energy particles. Prolonged exposure to this radiation can lead to severe health issues, including cancer, neurological damage, and acute radiation sickness [46]. Nanotechnology offers promising solutions for enhancing radiation protection through the development of advanced shielding materials and protective coatings. Nanomaterials such as boron nitride nanotubes (BNNTs) and hydrogen-rich nanocomposites are being explored for their ability to absorb or deflect harmful radiation. BNNTs, for example, have a high neutron absorption capacity, making them effective at reducing neutron radiation, a common component of cosmic rays [47]. Similarly, hydrogen-rich nanocomposites can shield against proton and heavy ion radiation, which are prevalent in space. These materials can be integrated into the spacecraft's hull, spacesuits, and other protective gear, providing a lightweight yet effective barrier against radiation. Moreover, nanotechnology enables the creation of adaptive or smart materials that can change their properties in response to varying levels of radiation [48]. These materials could adjust their radiation-blocking capabilities based on real-time exposure, offering more flexible and efficient protection. This adaptability is particularly useful for deep space missions, where radiation levels can fluctuate depending on solar activity or the spacecraft's proximity to different celestial bodies.

Nanotechnology in Satellite and Communication Systems

Nanotechnology is revolutionizing satellite and communication systems by improving the performance, durability, and efficiency of critical components. As global communication networks and space-based systems become increasingly important for both commercial and scientific applications, advancements in nanotechnology enable more reliable and efficient satellite operations [49]. This section explores two key areas where nanotechnology is making a significant impact: enhancing signal transmission with nano-antennas and improving energy harvesting through nano-coatings for solar panels. Nano-antennas, a breakthrough in nanotechnology, are designed to significantly improve signal transmission and reception in satellite communication systems. Unlike conventional antennas, which are often bulky and limited in performance, nano-antennas are composed of nanomaterials like carbon nanotubes and graphene that exhibit exceptional electrical properties [50]. These materials enable nano-antennas to operate at higher frequencies and transmit data at faster rates, which is crucial for modern communication systems that demand high bandwidth and low latency.

The small size of nano-antennas allows for more compact and lightweight satellite designs, which is particularly advantageous for small satellites or CubeSats, where space is at a premium, as illustrated in Fig. (**6.2**). Additionally, nano-antennas can be integrated into the surfaces of satellites or even deployed as part of flexible or foldable structures, maximizing their effectiveness while minimizing their footprint [51]. This miniaturization does not come at the cost of performance; in fact, nano-antennas can achieve higher gain and directivity, ensuring more reliable communication links between satellites and ground stations or between satellites in constellations. The use of nano-antennas allows for more sophisticated beamforming techniques, which can dynamically adjust the direction and focus of signals to improve communication accuracy and reduce interference. This is particularly important for deep space missions, where maintaining a stable and high-quality communication link over vast distances is challenging. The enhanced capabilities of nano-antennas ensure that satellites can transmit and receive signals more effectively, contributing to the overall reliability and efficiency of space-based communication networks [52].

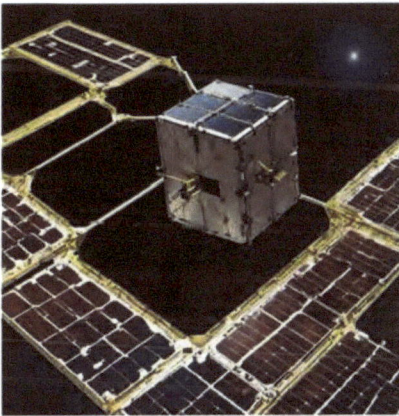

1. Cost-effective missions
2. Technology demonstration
3. Educational purposes
4. Earth observation
5. Scientific research

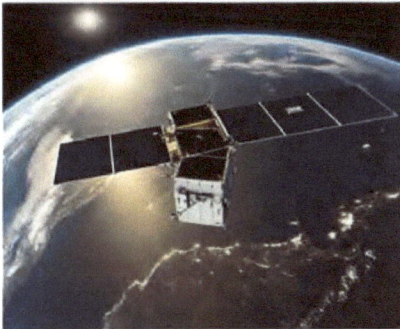

6. Communications support
7. Constellation deployment
8. Interplanetary missions
9. Quick deployment
10. Collaboration opportunities

Fig. (6.2). Role of nanosats and cubesats technology in satellite communications.

Energy harvesting is a critical aspect of satellite operation, especially for long-duration missions where power resources must be managed carefully. Solar panels are the primary source of energy for most satellites, converting sunlight into electrical power to support various onboard systems. However, traditional solar panels can suffer from degradation due to exposure to harsh space environments, including extreme temperatures, radiation, and micrometeoroid impacts. Nanotechnology addresses these challenges through the development of advanced nano-coatings that enhance the performance and longevity of solar panels [53]. Nano-coatings made from materials like titanium dioxide (TiO_2) and other nanocomposites provide multiple benefits. First, these coatings can improve the efficiency of solar panels by increasing their ability to capture and convert sunlight into electricity [54]. Nanostructured surfaces can reduce the reflection of sunlight and trap more photons, effectively boosting the energy output of the panels. This increase in efficiency is crucial for satellites, which rely on maximizing energy production to power their systems. Second, nano-coatings offer protective properties that extend the lifespan of solar panels. These coatings can provide resistance to radiation and thermal damage, reducing the wear and tear that solar panels typically experience in space. Additionally, nano-coatings can make solar panels more resistant to contamination from space debris and dust, which can degrade their performance over time. Some nano-coatings are even self-cleaning, repelling particles and ensuring that the panels remain clear and functional throughout the mission [55]. Nanotechnology also enables the development of flexible and lightweight solar panels that can be integrated into satellite structures more efficiently. These flexible panels, enhanced with nano-coatings, can be deployed in compact forms during launch and then expanded in space, providing larger surface areas for energy collection without adding significant weight to the satellite. This innovation not only improves the energy harvesting capabilities of satellites but also reduces the cost and complexity of deploying large solar arrays.

Nanotechnology in Space Propulsion Systems

Nanotechnology is significantly enhancing space propulsion systems by enabling more efficient, powerful, and sustainable propulsion methods. As space missions push the boundaries of exploration, from low Earth orbit to deep space, the need for advanced propulsion systems becomes paramount [56]. Nanotechnology contributes to this field by improving the performance of fuels and materials used in various propulsion systems, such as chemical rockets and ion thrusters. This section delves into the role of nano-fuels in boosting propulsion efficiency and the application of nanomaterials in ion thrusters for long-duration space travel. Nano-fuels represent a cutting-edge application of nanotechnology in chemical propulsion systems. These fuels incorporate nanoparticles into traditional propellants, enhancing their combustion properties and overall efficiency [57]. The addition of nanoparticles, such as aluminum or boron-based particles, can significantly increase the energy density of the fuel. This results in a higher thrust-to-weight ratio, which is crucial for overcoming the immense gravitational pull during a spacecraft's launch and for maneuvers in space. The smaller particle size in nano-fuels allows for more uniform and rapid combustion, reducing fuel consumption while delivering the same or even greater amounts of energy. This efficiency is particularly valuable for missions where fuel mass is a critical constraint. By using nano-fuels, spacecraft can carry less fuel for the same mission profile, reducing launch costs and increasing the payload capacity [58]. Additionally, nano-fuels can be engineered to produce less toxic byproducts and have higher stability, which enhances the safety and environmental friendliness of space missions. The versatility of nano-fuels extends to their adaptability in various propulsion systems, from solid rockets to hybrid engines. This flexibility allows for more customized propulsion solutions tailored to specific mission needs, whether for launching satellites into orbit or propelling spacecraft on interplanetary journeys.

Ion thrusters, a form of electric propulsion, have become increasingly important for long-duration space missions due to their high efficiency and ability to provide continuous thrust over extended periods. Nanotechnology is revolutionizing ion thrusters by improving the materials used in their construction, leading to better performance and longevity. Nanomaterials such as carbon nanotubes, graphene, and advanced ceramics are being integrated into various components of ion thrusters to enhance their capabilities [59]. One of the key challenges in ion thrusters is managing the wear and erosion of critical components, such as the grids that accelerate ions. Nanomaterials offer superior resistance to erosion and high temperatures, which are common issues in ion thrusters. For example, carbon nanotubes and graphene-based coatings can be applied to the thruster grids, significantly reducing wear and prolonging the operational life of the thruster. This durability is essential for missions that require propulsion over several years, such as deep space probes or interplanetary missions. In addition to durability, nanomaterials can improve the overall efficiency of ion thrusters. The enhanced electrical conductivity of nanomaterials enables better ionization of the propellant, resulting in higher thrust levels with the same amount of fuel [60]. This increased efficiency reduces the amount of propellant needed, allowing spacecraft to travel farther with less mass. Nanotechnology also enables the development of lighter and more compact ion thrusters, which can be integrated into smaller spacecraft or used as part of multi-thruster arrays for more powerful propulsion systems. The use of nanomaterials in ion thrusters opens the door to innovative designs, such as flexible or deployable thrusters, which can be folded during launch and deployed in space [61]. These designs allow for greater adaptability in spacecraft configurations and mission profiles, providing more options for maneuvering and propulsion in different space environments.

CHALLENGES AND OPPORTUNITIES

Nanotechnology holds immense potential for space exploration, but several challenges must be addressed to fully realize its benefits. The successful integration of nanotechnology into space missions requires overcoming obstacles related to manufacturing and scalability, as well as ensuring the durability and reliability of nanomaterials in the harsh conditions of space. One of the primary challenges in implementing nanotechnology in space missions is the complexity of manufacturing and scaling up nanomaterials for practical use [62]. While laboratory-scale production of nanomaterials like carbon nanotubes, graphene, and nano-composites has shown promising results, transitioning these materials to large-scale production suitable for spacecraft components remains a significant hurdle. The precision required in nanomaterial fabrication makes mass production costly and time-consuming, which limits the widespread adoption of these materials in space exploration. The quality and consistency of nanomaterials produced at scale can be difficult to maintain. Variations in material properties can affect the performance and safety of spacecraft, making it crucial to develop reliable and reproducible manufacturing processes [63]. As a result, research is ongoing to refine fabrication techniques and develop cost-effective methods for producing high-quality nanomaterials at scale. Addressing these issues is essential for making nanotechnology a viable option for space missions, where reliability and performance are critical.

Space presents an exceptionally harsh environment, with extreme temperatures, radiation, and the vacuum of space posing significant challenges to the durability and reliability of materials. Nanomaterials, while offering remarkable properties in controlled environments, must be rigorously tested and optimized for use in space. Ensuring that these materials can withstand the stresses of launch, prolonged exposure to cosmic radiation, and thermal cycling between the intense heat of the sun and the cold of deep space is critical [64]. For example, while carbon nanotubes and graphene are known for their strength and conductivity, their behavior under space conditions must be thoroughly understood. Issues such as radiation-induced degradation, thermal expansion, and the effects of prolonged exposure to vacuum environments can impact their performance. Ensuring the long-term stability and reliability of nanomaterials in space requires extensive testing and material engineering, which can be both time-consuming and costly. Another challenge is the potential for nanomaterials to interact with the unique conditions of space in unexpected ways [65]. For instance, nanoparticles might agglomerate or behave differently in microgravity, affecting their intended functions. These challenges underscore the need for thorough testing and the development of robust designs that can ensure the reliability of nanotechnology in space missions.

Despite the challenges, the opportunities presented by nanotechnology for space exploration are vast. Innovations in nanomaterials and their applications, coupled with collaboration between space agencies and nanotechnology experts, hold the promise of transforming future space missions. The continuous innovation in nanomaterials is opening new possibilities for space exploration. Research in advanced nanomaterials, such as ultra-lightweight aerogels, self-healing materials, and multifunctional nano-coatings, is expanding the range of applications for nanotechnology in space. These innovations have the potential to improve spacecraft design, making them more efficient, durable, and capable of withstanding the rigors of space travel. For example, the development of self-healing nanomaterials could enable spacecraft to repair themselves in the event of damage from micrometeoroids or space debris, enhancing mission safety and longevity [66]. Similarly, the creation of nanomaterials with enhanced radiation shielding capabilities could protect astronauts and sensitive equipment from harmful cosmic rays, a critical consideration for long-duration missions to destinations like Mars [67]. In addition to material innovations, advancements in nanoelectronics and nano-sensors are paving the way for more sophisticated and miniaturized space instruments. These technologies can enable more precise measurements, more efficient data processing, and reduced power consumption, all of which are crucial for deep space exploration and autonomous spacecraft. The successful integration of nanotechnology into space missions requires collaboration between space agencies, academic institutions, and nanotechnology experts. By fostering partnerships across disciplines, space agencies can leverage the latest advancements in nanotechnology to address specific challenges in space exploration. This collaboration is essential for developing new technologies, testing them under space conditions, and refining them for practical use in missions. For instance, collaborations between NASA and research institutions have already led to significant breakthroughs in nanomaterials for space applications [68]. Joint efforts between space agencies and nanotechnology companies can accelerate the development of next-generation spacecraft materials and systems. Furthermore, international collaborations can pool resources and expertise, ensuring that the benefits of nanotechnology are realized on a global scale. These partnerships also open opportunities for funding and research grants, which can drive further innovation in the field. By working together, space agencies and nanotechnology experts can overcome the current challenges and unlock the full potential of nanotechnology for space exploration, enabling more ambitious missions and advancing humanity's reach into the cosmos.

CONCLUSION

Nanotechnology has emerged as a transformative force in space exploration, fundamentally altering the way we design spacecraft, conduct missions, and envision the future of space travel. The integration of nanomaterials into spacecraft design has led to significant advancements in reducing weight while enhancing strength and durability, allowing for more efficient and resilient spacecraft. Nano-sensors and instruments have revolutionized data collection and analysis, offering increased sensitivity, precision, and energy efficiency. Additionally, nanotechnology has opened new frontiers in deep space exploration, providing solutions for long-duration missions and radiation protection, and enhancing satellite and communication systems through innovations like nano-antennas and advanced solar coatings. Nanotechnology has enabled more ambitious and cost-effective missions, making space exploration more accessible and pushing the boundaries of what is possible in the cosmos. Looking ahead, the future of nanotechnology in space exploration is filled with exciting possibilities and potential breakthroughs. Continued research and development in nanomaterials are expected to yield even more advanced materials with multifunctional properties, such as self-healing capabilities, superior radiation shielding, and ultra-lightweight structures. Innovations in nanoelectronics, quantum dots, and nanosensors will further enhance spacecraft capabilities, enabling more autonomous and intelligent missions. As space agencies and nanotechnology experts collaborate more closely, we can anticipate breakthroughs in propulsion systems, energy harvesting, and *in-situ* resource utilization, which will be critical for long-term space habitation and interplanetary travel. The growing commercialization of space may drive the development of new nano-enabled technologies, making space exploration more sustainable and economically viable. Ultimately, nanotechnology will continue to play a pivotal role in shaping the future of space exploration, enabling humanity to explore deeper into the universe and realize the dream of becoming a multi-planetary species.

REFERENCES

[1]   Donaldson, L. Stacked 2D nanomeshes that offer unique physical properties. *Mater. Today,* **2021**, *47*, 2.
        [http://dx.doi.org/10.1016/j.mattod.2021.06.010]

[2]   Liang, M.; Yan, X. Nanozymes: From New Concepts, Mechanisms, and Standards to Applications. *Acc. Chem. Res.,* **2019**, *52*(8), 2190-2200.
        [http://dx.doi.org/10.1021/acs.accounts.9b00140] [PMID: 31276379]

[3]   Wang, Z.L.; Song, J. Piezoelectric nanogenerators based on zinc oxide nanowire arrays. *Science,* **2006**, *312*(5771), 242-246.
        [http://dx.doi.org/10.1126/science.1124005] [PMID: 16614215]

[4]   Gramotnev, D.K.; Bozhevolnyi, S.I. Plasmonics beyond the diffraction limit. *Nat. Photonics,* **2010**,

4(2), 83-91.
[http://dx.doi.org/10.1038/nphoton.2009.282]

[5]   Aricò, A.S.; Bruce, P.; Scrosati, B.; Tarascon, J.M.; van Schalkwijk, W. Nanostructured materials for advanced energy conversion and storage devices. *Nat. Mater.,* **2005**, *4*(5), 366-377.
[http://dx.doi.org/10.1038/nmat1368] [PMID: 15867920]

[6]   Simon, P.; Gogotsi, Y. Capacitive energy storage in nanostructured carbon-electrolyte systems. *Acc. Chem. Res.,* **2013**, *46*(5), 1094-1103.
[http://dx.doi.org/10.1021/ar200306b] [PMID: 22670843]

[7]   Grotzinger, J.P.; Crisp, J.; Vasavada, A.R.; Anderson, R.C.; Baker, C.J.; Barry, R.; Blake, D.F.; Conrad, P.; Edgett, K.S.; Ferdowski, B.; Gellert, R.; Gilbert, J.B.; Golombek, M.; Gómez-Elvira, J.; Hassler, D.M.; Jandura, L.; Litvak, M.; Mahaffy, P.; Maki, J.; Meyer, M.; Malin, M.C.; Mitrofanov, I.; Simmonds, J.J.; Vaniman, D.; Welch, R.V.; Wiens, R.C. Mars science laboratory mission and science investigation. *Space Sci. Rev.,* **2012**, *170*(1-4), 5-56.
[http://dx.doi.org/10.1007/s11214-012-9892-2]

[8]   Frampton, W.J.; Dash, J.; Watmough, G.; Milton, E.J. Evaluating the capabilities of Sentinel-2 for quantitative estimation of biophysical variables in vegetation. *ISPRS J. Photogramm. Remote Sens.,* **2013**, *82*, 83-92.
[http://dx.doi.org/10.1016/j.isprsjprs.2013.04.007]

[9]   Guo, Y. Solar Probe Plus: Mission design challenges and trades. *Acta Astronaut.,* **2010**, *67*(9-10), 1063-1072.
[http://dx.doi.org/10.1016/j.actaastro.2010.06.007]

[10]   Mori, O. A1 world's first solar power sail demonstration flight by IKAROS. *The Proceedings of the Space Engineering Conference,* **2011**, *19* (1), 1-7.
[http://dx.doi.org/10.1299/jsmesec.2010.19._A1-1_]

[11]   Boley, A.C.; Byers, M. Satellite mega-constellations create risks in Low Earth Orbit, the atmosphere and on Earth. *Sci. Rep.,* **2021**, *11*(1), 10642.
[http://dx.doi.org/10.1038/s41598-021-89909-7] [PMID: 34017017]

[12]   Carlson, L.J.; Krauss, T.D. Photophysics of individual single-walled carbon nanotubes. *Acc. Chem. Res.,* **2008**, *41*(2), 235-243.
[http://dx.doi.org/10.1021/ar700136v] [PMID: 18281946]

[13]   Varadan, V.K.; Xie, J. Large-scale synthesis of multi-walled carbon nanotubes by microwave CVD. *Smart Mater. Struct.,* **2002**, *11*(4), 610-616.
[http://dx.doi.org/10.1088/0964-1726/11/4/318]

[14]   Shahil, K.M.F.; Balandin, A.A. Thermal properties of graphene and multilayer graphene: Applications in thermal interface materials. *Solid State Commun.,* **2012**, *152*(15), 1331-1340.
[http://dx.doi.org/10.1016/j.ssc.2012.04.034]

[15]   Patra, J.K.; Das, G.; Fraceto, L.F.; Campos, E.V.R.; Rodriguez-Torres, M.P.; Acosta-Torres, L.S.; Diaz-Torres, L.A.; Grillo, R.; Swamy, M.K.; Sharma, S.; Habtemariam, S.; Shin, H.S. Nano based drug delivery systems: recent developments and future prospects. *J. Nanobiotechnology,* **2018**, *16*(1), 71.
[http://dx.doi.org/10.1186/s12951-018-0392-8] [PMID: 30231877]

[16]   Warheit, D.; Hoke, R.; Finlay, C.; Donner, E.; Reed, K.; Sayes, C. Development of a base set of toxicity tests using ultrafine TiO_2 particles as a component of nanoparticle risk management. *Toxicol. Lett.,* **2007**, *171*(3), 99-110.
[http://dx.doi.org/10.1016/j.toxlet.2007.04.008] [PMID: 17566673]

[17]   Rasul, M. G.; Kiziltas, A.; Arfaei, B.; Shahbazian-Yassar, R. 2D Boron Nitride Nanosheets for Polymer Composite Materials. *NPJ 2D Materials and Applications,* **2021**, *5*(1).
[http://dx.doi.org/10.1038/s41699-021-00231-2]

[18]   Baker, S.N.; Baker, G.A. Luminescent carbon nanodots: emergent nanolights. *Angew. Chem. Int. Ed.,* **2010**, *49*(38), 6726-6744.
[http://dx.doi.org/10.1002/anie.200906623] [PMID: 20687055]

[19]   Jo, S.; Kim, T.; Im, W. Automated builder and database of protein/membrane complexes for molecular dynamics simulations. *PLoS One,* **2007**, *2*(9), e880.
[http://dx.doi.org/10.1371/journal.pone.0000880] [PMID: 17849009]

[20]   Kalakonda, P.; Banne, S.; Kalakonda, P.B. Enhanced mechanical properties of multiwalled carbon nanotubes/thermoplastic polyurethane nanocomposites. *Nanomaterials and Nanotechnology,* **2019**, *9*.
[http://dx.doi.org/10.1177/1847980419840858]

[21]   Qu, X.; Alvarez, P.J.J.; Li, Q. Applications of nanotechnology in water and wastewater treatment. *Water Res.,* **2013**, *47*(12), 3931-3946.
[http://dx.doi.org/10.1016/j.watres.2012.09.058] [PMID: 23571110]

[22]   Zheng, J.Y.; Yan, Y.; Wang, X.; Shi, W.; Ma, H.; Zhao, Y.S.; Yao, J. Hydrogen peroxide vapor sensing with organic core/sheath nanowire optical waveguides. *Adv. Mater.,* **2012**, *24*(35), OP194-OP199, OP186.
[http://dx.doi.org/10.1002/adma.201200867] [PMID: 22760953]

[23]   Matthes, C.; Stumbo, M.; Foley, J.; Dang, T. Jose Trujillo Rojas. How to build a rover: An overview of the mars 2020 mission's vehicle system testbed. *IEEE Aerospace Conference (AERO),* **2022**.
[http://dx.doi.org/10.1109/AERO53065.2022.9843658]

[24]   Soja, R.H.; Altobelli, N.; Krüger, H.; Sterken, V.J. Dust environment predictions for the ESA L-class mission JUICE. *Planet. Space Sci.,* **2013**, *75*, 117-128.
[http://dx.doi.org/10.1016/j.pss.2012.11.010]

[25]   Smith, M.; Craig, D.; Herrmann, N.; Mahoney, E.; Krezel, J.; McIntyre, N.; Goodliff, K. The Artemis Program: An Overview of NASA's Activities to Return Humans to the Moon. *2020 IEEE Aerospace Conference, Big Sky, MT, USA,,* **2020**, 1-10.
[http://dx.doi.org/10.1109/AERO47225.2020.9172323]

[26]   Kumar, M. Interpreted investigation report: Loss of vikram lander during lunar landing phase. **2023**.

[27]   Li, X. Friso van Amerom; Graham, J. D.; Andrej Grubisic; Francom, M. B.; Barfknecht, P. W.; Brinckerhoff, W. B.; Trainer, M. G.; Castillo, M. E. Laser Desorption Mass Spectrometry of Cryogenic Samples on the Dragonfly Mission. *IEEE Aerospace Conference,* **2023**.
[http://dx.doi.org/10.1109/AERO55745.2023.10115534]

[28]   Josef, S.; Degani, A. Deep Reinforcement Learning for Safe Local Planning of a Ground Vehicle in Unknown Rough Terrain. *IEEE Robot. Autom. Lett.,* **2020**, *5*(4), 6748-6755.
[http://dx.doi.org/10.1109/LRA.2020.3011912]

[29]   Vm, A. Gas and Biosensors Made from Metal Oxides Doped with Carbon Nanotubes. *Physical Science & Biophysics Journal,* **2021**, *5*(1).
[http://dx.doi.org/10.23880/psbj-16000176]

[30]   Duncan, T.V. Applications of nanotechnology in food packaging and food safety: Barrier materials, antimicrobials and sensors. *J. Colloid Interface Sci.,* **2011**, *363*(1), 1-24.
[http://dx.doi.org/10.1016/j.jcis.2011.07.017] [PMID: 21824625]

[31]   Pratx, G.; Carpenter, C.M.; Sun, C.; Xing, L. X-ray luminescence computed tomography *via* selective excitation: a feasibility study. *IEEE Trans. Med. Imaging,* **2010**, *29*(12), 1992-1999.
[http://dx.doi.org/10.1109/TMI.2010.2055883] [PMID: 20615807]

[32]   Qin, J.; Jiang, S.; Wang, Z.; Cheng, X.; Li, B.; Shi, Y.; Tsai, D.P.; Liu, A.Q.; Huang, W.; Zhu, W. Metasurface Micro/Nano-Optical Sensors: Principles and Applications. *ACS Nano,* **2022**, *16*(8), 11598-11618.
[http://dx.doi.org/10.1021/acsnano.2c03310] [PMID: 35960685]

[33] de Haan, S. NEMS—emerging products and applications of nano-electromechanical systems. *Nanotechnol. Percept.,* **2006**, *2*(3), 267-275.
[http://dx.doi.org/10.4024/N14HA06.ntp.02.03]

[34] Zhu, S.; Song, Y.; Zhao, X.; Shao, J.; Zhang, J.; Yang, B. The photoluminescence mechanism in carbon dots (graphene quantum dots, carbon nanodots, and polymer dots): current state and future perspective. *Nano Res.,* **2015**, *8*(2), 355-381.
[http://dx.doi.org/10.1007/s12274-014-0644-3]

[35] Kim, D.; Chung, N.K.; Allen, S.; Tendler, S.J.B.; Park, J.W. Ferritin-based new magnetic force microscopic probe detecting 10 nm sized magnetic nanoparticles. *ACS Nano,* **2012**, *6*(1), 241-248.
[http://dx.doi.org/10.1021/nn203464g] [PMID: 22148318]

[36] Dorozhkin, S.V. Calcium orthophosphate-based biocomposites and hybrid biomaterials. *J. Mater. Sci.,* **2009**, *44*(9), 2343-2387.
[http://dx.doi.org/10.1007/s10853-008-3124-x]

[37] Khan, Z.H.; Kermany, A.R.; Öchsner, A.; Iacopi, F. Mechanical and electromechanical properties of graphene and their potential application in MEMS. *J. Phys. D Appl. Phys.,* **2017**, *50*(5), 053003.
[http://dx.doi.org/10.1088/1361-6463/50/5/053003]

[38] Blakey-Milner, B.; Gradl, P.; Snedden, G.; Brooks, M.; Pitot, J.; Lopez, E.; Leary, M.; Berto, F.; du Plessis, A. Metal additive manufacturing in aerospace: A review. *Mater. Des.,* **2021**, *209*(1), 110008.
[http://dx.doi.org/10.1016/j.matdes.2021.110008]

[39] Bonaccorso, F.; Sun, Z.; Hasan, T.; Ferrari, A.C. Graphene photonics and optoelectronics. *Nat. Photonics,* **2010**, *4*(9), 611-622.
[http://dx.doi.org/10.1038/nphoton.2010.186]

[40] Lu, S.Y.; Mukhopadhyay, S.; Froese, R.; Zimmerman, P.M. Virtual Screening of Hole Transport, Electron Transport, and Host Layers for Effective OLED Design. *J. Chem. Inf. Model.,* **2018**, *58*(12), 2440-2449.
[http://dx.doi.org/10.1021/acs.jcim.8b00044] [PMID: 29949358]

[41] Li, X.; Yao, H.; Wang, J.; Xu, X.; Jiang, C.; Hanzo, L. A Near-Optimal UAV-Aided Radio Coverage Strategy for Dense Urban Areas. *IEEE Trans. Vehicular Technol.,* **2019**, *68*(9), 9098-9109.
[http://dx.doi.org/10.1109/TVT.2019.2927425]

[42] Clifton, T.; Ferreira, P.G.; Padilla, A.; Skordis, C. Modified gravity and cosmology. *Phys. Rep.,* **2012**, 513(1), 1–189.
[http://dx.doi.org/10.1016/j.physrep.2012.01.001]

[43] *Vision and Voyages for Planetary Science in the Decade 2013-2022*; National Academies Press: Washington, D.C., **2011**.
[http://dx.doi.org/10.17226/13117]

[44] Richardson, T. Spinal column and midbrain integration for long duration space missions. *F1000 Res.,* **2023**, *12*, 946-946.
[http://dx.doi.org/10.12688/f1000research.129719.1]

[45] Sharma, V.K.; Yngard, R.A.; Lin, Y. Silver nanoparticles: Green synthesis and their antimicrobial activities. *Adv. Colloid Interface Sci.,* **2009**, *145*(1-2), 83-96.
[http://dx.doi.org/10.1016/j.cis.2008.09.002] [PMID: 18945421]

[46] Okunewick, J.P.; Hartley, K.M.; Darden, J. Comparison of radiation sensitivity, endogenous colony formation, and erythropoietin response following prolonged hypoxia exposure. *Radiat. Res.,* **1969**, *38*(3), 530-543.
[http://dx.doi.org/10.2307/3572612] [PMID: 5790118]

[47] Silva, W.M.; Ribeiro, H.; Taha-Tijerina, J.J. Potential Production of Theranostic Boron Nitride Nanotubes (^{64}Cu-BNNTs) Radiolabeled by Neutron Capture. *Nanomaterials (Basel),* **2021**, *11*(11), 2907.

[http://dx.doi.org/10.3390/nano11112907] [PMID: 34835671]

[48]   Owen, R.; Macnaghten, P.; Stilgoe, J. Responsible research and innovation: From science in society to science for society, with society. *Sci. Public Policy,* **2012**, *39*(6), 751-760.
[http://dx.doi.org/10.1093/scipol/scs093]

[49]   Levchenko, I.; Bazaka, K.; Ding, Y.; Raitses, Y.; Mazouffre, S.; Henning, T.; Klar, P.J.; Shinohara, S.; Schein, J.; Garrigues, L.; Kim, M.; Lev, D.; Taccogna, F.; Boswell, R.W.; Charles, C.; Koizumi, H.; Shen, Y.; Scharlemann, C.; Keidar, M.; Xu, S. Space micropropulsion systems for Cubesats and small satellites: From proximate targets to furthermost frontiers. *Appl. Phys. Rev.,* **2018**, *5*(1), 011104.
[http://dx.doi.org/10.1063/1.5007734]

[50]   Larsson, E.G.; Edfors, O.; Tufvesson, F.; Marzetta, T.L. Massive MIMO for next generation wireless systems. *IEEE Commun. Mag.,* **2014**, *52*(2), 186-195.
[http://dx.doi.org/10.1109/MCOM.2014.6736761]

[51]   Zhou, F.; Liu, Y.; Li, Z.Y.; Xia, Y. Analytical model for optical bistability in nonlinear metal nano-antennae involving Kerr materials. *Opt. Express,* **2010**, *18*(13), 13337-13344.
[http://dx.doi.org/10.1364/OE.18.013337] [PMID: 20588463]

[52]   Tariq, F.; Khandaker, M.R.A.; Wong, K.K.; Imran, M.A.; Bennis, M.; Debbah, M. A Speculative Study on 6G. *IEEE Wirel. Commun.,* **2020**, *27*(4), 118-125.
[http://dx.doi.org/10.1109/MWC.001.1900488]

[53]   Dakal, T.C.; Kumar, A.; Majumdar, R.S.; Yadav, V. Mechanistic basis of antimicrobial actions of silver nanoparticles. *Front. Microbiol.,* **2016**, *7*, 1831.
[http://dx.doi.org/10.3389/fmicb.2016.01831] [PMID: 27899918]

[54]   Graphene Coating Promises to Improve Condenser Efficiency. *Focus on Powder Coatings,* **2015**, *2015*(8), 5.
[http://dx.doi.org/10.1016/j.fopow.2015.07.025]

[55]   Eshaghi, A. Transparent hard self-cleaning nano-hybrid coating on polymeric substrate. *Prog. Org. Coat.,* **2019**, *128*, 120-126.
[http://dx.doi.org/10.1016/j.porgcoat.2018.12.021]

[56]   Chandra, S. Indian Space Exploration: Economic Missions and Global Comparisons. *Open Access Journal of Astronomy,* **2024**, *2*(2), 1-3.
[http://dx.doi.org/10.23880/oaja-16000126]

[57]   Sugioka, K.; Cheng, Y. Ultrafast lasers—reliable tools for advanced materials processing. *Light Sci. Appl.,* **2014**, *3*(4), e149-e149.
[http://dx.doi.org/10.1038/lsa.2014.30]

[58]   Middleton, D.B.; Hurt, G.J., Jr Lunar E cape-to-Orbit Systems Simulation (LESS) Using Simplified Manual Control. *J. Spacecr. Rockets,* **1971**, *8*(10), 1011-1017.
[http://dx.doi.org/10.2514/3.59762]

[59]   Dai, L.; Chang, D.W.; Baek, J.B.; Lu, W. Carbon nanomaterials for advanced energy conversion and storage. *Small,* **2012**, *8*(8), 1130-1166.
[http://dx.doi.org/10.1002/smll.201101594] [PMID: 22383334]

[60]   Huang, M.H.; Rej, S.; Hsu, S.C. Facet-dependent properties of polyhedral nanocrystals. *Chem. Commun. (Camb.),* **2014**, *50*(14), 1634-1644.
[http://dx.doi.org/10.1039/c3cc48527g] [PMID: 24406546]

[61]   Bheekhun, N.; Abu Talib, A.R.; Hassan, M.R. Aerogels in Aerospace: An Overview. *Adv. Mater. Sci. Eng.,* **2013**, *2013*, 1-18.
[http://dx.doi.org/10.1155/2013/406065]

[62]   Amadei, C.A.; Montessori, A.; Kadow, J.P.; Succi, S.; Vecitis, C.D. Role of oxygen functionalities in graphene oxide architectural laminate subnanometer spacing and water transport. *Environ. Sci. Technol.,* **2017**, *51*(8), 4280-4288.

[http://dx.doi.org/10.1021/acs.est.6b05711] [PMID: 28333448]

[63]   Cummer, S.A.; Popa, B.I.; Schurig, D.; Smith, D.R.; Pendry, J. Full-wave simulations of electromagnetic cloaking structures. *Phys. Rev. E Stat. Nonlin. Soft Matter Phys.,* **2006**, *74*(3), 036621. [http://dx.doi.org/10.1103/PhysRevE.74.036621] [PMID: 17025778]

[64]   Koops, L. Cosmic Radiation Exposure of Future Hypersonic Flight Missions. *Radiat. Prot. Dosimetry,* **2017**, *175*(2), 267-278. [http://dx.doi.org/10.1093/rpd/ncw298] [PMID: 27886995]

[65]   Steffen, W.; Richardson, K.; Rockström, J.; Cornell, S.E.; Fetzer, I.; Bennett, E.M.; Biggs, R.; Carpenter, S.R.; de Vries, W.; de Wit, C.A.; Folke, C.; Gerten, D.; Heinke, J.; Mace, G.M.; Persson, L.M.; Ramanathan, V.; Reyers, B.; Sörlin, S. Planetary boundaries: Guiding human development on a changing planet. *Science,* **2015**, *347*(6223), 1259855. [http://dx.doi.org/10.1126/science.1259855] [PMID: 25592418]

[66]   Li, Q. Albertus; Bunning, T. J. *Light-Responsive Smart Soft Matter Technologies.,* **2019**, *7*(16), 1901160-1901160. [http://dx.doi.org/10.1002/adom.201901160]

[67]   Cheraghi, E.; Chen, S.; Yeow, J.T.W. Boron Nitride-Based Nanomaterials for Radiation Shielding: A Review. *IEEE Nanotechnol. Mag.,* **2021**, *15*(3), 8-17. [http://dx.doi.org/10.1109/MNANO.2021.3066390]

[68]   Dennison, J.R. Dynamic Interplay Between Spacecraft Charging, Space Environment Interactions, and Evolving Materials. *IEEE Trans. Plasma Sci.,* **2015**, *43*(9), 2933-2940. [http://dx.doi.org/10.1109/TPS.2015.2434947]

CHAPTER 7

Nanotechnology in Art and Cultural Heritage

Abstract: Nanotechnology, with its ability to manipulate materials at the molecular and atomic levels, is revolutionizing the fields of art and cultural heritage. This chapter explores the multifaceted role of nanotechnology in the preservation, restoration, and creation of art. The use of nanomaterials and nano-coatings has shown significant promise in preventing the deterioration of historical sites, artworks, and monuments, with successful implementations. Nanotechnology offers advanced methods for cleaning and structurally reinforcing artifacts, including paintings and sculptures. The use of nanocomposites and other nanoscale materials allows for precise and effective interventions that preserve the integrity of the original work while extending its lifespan. This chapter discusses the emerging field of nano-art, where artists harness the unique properties of nanomaterials to create innovative and interactive art forms. The exploration of these new media showcases the potential for nanotechnology to redefine artistic expression in the 21st century. However, the role of nanotechnology in art and cultural heritage also raises ethical concerns. Balancing innovation with tradition, ensuring authenticity, and mitigating potential risks are critical challenges that must be addressed. The ethical implications of altering historical artifacts with modern technology, as well as the long-term effects of such interventions, require careful consideration. This chapter looks to the future, envisioning the continued convergence of nanotechnology and art. Emerging art forms and the ongoing development of nanomaterials promise to further blur the lines between science and creativity.

Keywords: Cultural heritage, Nano-art, Nanocomposites, Preservation, Restoration, UV radiation.

INTRODUCTION

Nanotechnology, often described as the science of manipulating matter at the nanometer scale (one billionth of a meter), is revolutionizing various fields, including medicine, electronics, and environmental science [1]. In recent years, its application in art and cultural heritage has emerged as a groundbreaking area of research and practice. Art and cultural heritage encompass a vast range of objects, from ancient manuscripts and paintings to architectural monuments and archaeological artifacts. These items are not just physical objects; they are carriers of history, culture, and identity [2]. However, they are often vulnerable to deterioration due to factors like aging, environmental exposure, human handling,

Shivang Dhoundiyal & Aftab Alam

and previous restoration efforts. Traditional conservation methods have sometimes been inadequate in addressing these challenges, often due to their invasive nature or limitations in reversing damage without altering the artifact. Nanotechnology offers a promising alternative by enabling the manipulation of materials at the molecular level, thus providing unprecedented control over the preservation process. The small size of nanoparticles allows them to interact with the surface and interior of artifacts in highly specific ways [3]. For instance, nanoparticles can be engineered to bond with the materials in a painting or sculpture, strengthening them without adding bulk or altering the original appearance. This ability to interact on such a fine scale allows for precise cleaning, stabilization, and protection of delicate artifacts. Moreover, nanotechnology is not just confined to the preservation of existing works; it also opens up new possibilities for artistic creation. Artists are beginning to experiment with nanomaterials to produce colors and effects that were previously impossible, giving rise to a new genre of "nano-art [4]." By leveraging the properties of nanotechnology, artists can create works that challenge traditional notions of form, texture, and color, expanding the boundaries of artistic expression.

The significance of nanotechnology in the preservation and restoration of cultural heritage cannot be overstated. The traditional methods of conservation, while historically valuable, often fall short when dealing with modern challenges, such as pollution, climate change, and the inevitable wear and tear that comes with time [5]. Nanotechnology introduces a set of tools that are more precise, effective, and minimally invasive. One of the most important applications of nanotechnology in preservation is the development of nano-coatings. These ultra-thin, transparent layers can be applied to the surface of artworks, manuscripts, and monuments to protect them from external damage without altering their appearance [6]. For example, nano-coatings can repel water, block harmful ultraviolet rays, and even prevent the growth of mold or bacteria. These properties make nano-coatings an essential tool in extending the lifespan of culturally significant objects. In addition to protection, nanotechnology plays a crucial role in the restoration of damaged or deteriorated artifacts [7]. Traditional restoration techniques, such as the application of solvents to clean a painting, can be harsh and may sometimes cause further damage. Nanotechnology provides a gentler approach. For example, nanomaterials can be engineered to selectively remove contaminants, such as dirt, oils, or old varnish layers, without affecting the underlying original material. This level of precision is particularly important when dealing with fragile objects that cannot withstand the stress of traditional cleaning methods. Furthermore, nanotechnology enables the reinforcement of weakened structures [8]. For example, in the case of a crumbling fresco or a fragile manuscript, nanoparticles can be used to penetrate deep into the material, filling microscopic cracks and voids, thus restoring the structural integrity of the object without adding weight or altering its appearance. The importance of nanotechnology extends beyond individual artifacts to entire architectural structures and historical sites [9]. Nanomaterials are being used to reinforce building materials, such as stone and mortar, making them more resistant to environmental degradation. This is particularly valuable in the preservation of ancient monuments that are exposed to harsh weather conditions and pollution. By stabilizing these structures at the molecular level, nanotechnology helps to preserve not just the physical integrity of these sites but also their cultural and historical significance. The role of nanotechnology in art and cultural heritage is not limited to conservation and restoration [10]. It is also a powerful tool for research and analysis. Advanced nanotechnology-based imaging techniques, such as atomic force microscopy and scanning electron microscopy, allow scientists to study the composition and structure of artworks and artifacts with incredible detail. This can provide valuable insights into the materials and techniques used by artists and craftsmen of the past, helping to inform more accurate and respectful restoration practices.

NANOTECHNOLOGY IN PRESERVATION TECHNIQUES

Nanomaterials, due to their unique properties at the atomic and molecular levels, have revolutionized the way we approach the preservation of cultural heritage. Traditional materials and methods often fall short in preventing the degradation of artifacts, especially those that are exposed to environmental stressors like humidity, pollution, ultraviolet (UV) radiation, and temperature fluctuations [11]. Nanomaterials, however, offer a more effective solution due to their small size, large surface area, and ability to interact at a molecular level with the materials that make up these artifacts. For example, nanoparticles of calcium hydroxide have been used to reinforce and stabilize deteriorating paper, frescoes, and other porous materials by penetrating deep into their structure and reacting with carbon dioxide to form calcium carbonate, which strengthens the material from within [12]. Similarly, nanoparticles can be used to neutralize acidic conditions that often lead to the decay of paper or textiles, thereby preventing further degradation. In addition, nanomaterials can be engineered to mimic the properties of original materials, enabling restorers to reinforce artifacts without altering their appearance or historical integrity [13]. The ability to design nanoparticles that can bond with specific materials means that conservators can create customized solutions tailored to the unique needs of each artifact, ensuring more effective and long-lasting preservation, as mentioned in Table **7.1**.

Nano-coatings represent a significant advancement in the protection of artworks and monuments, as depicted in Fig. (**7.1**). These ultra-thin layers, often only a few nanometers thick, can provide a powerful barrier against environmental damage while being completely invisible to the naked eye [14]. This is particularly important in preserving the aesthetic and historical value of artifacts, as traditional protective coatings can sometimes alter the appearance or texture of a piece. Nano-coatings are typically composed of materials such as titanium dioxide, silica, or carbon-based compounds, which have been engineered to provide specific protective functions [15]. For example, titanium dioxide nanoparticles are known for their photocatalytic properties, meaning they can break down organic pollutants when exposed to light, thus keeping surfaces clean and free from harmful substances [16]. This self-cleaning ability is especially valuable for outdoor monuments and statues, which are constantly exposed to pollutants from the atmosphere. Additionally, nano-coatings can be hydrophobic, meaning they repel water and prevent moisture from penetrating the surface of the artifact. This is crucial in preventing water-related damage, such as corrosion in metal objects or the growth of mold and mildew in porous materials like stone or wood [17]. Nano-coatings can provide protection against UV radiation, which is one of the primary causes of fading and deterioration in artworks, especially those that involve pigments and dyes. By blocking or reflecting UV rays, these coatings help maintain the vibrancy and integrity of colors over time. This is particularly important for outdoor sculptures, murals, and historical buildings that are exposed to sunlight. The durability and longevity of nano-coatings also mean that they require less frequent reapplication compared to traditional coatings, reducing the need for ongoing maintenance and minimizing the risk of damage during the preservation process [18]. Another innovative application of nano-coatings is in preventing biological degradation. Many historical artifacts and monuments are vulnerable to attack by microorganisms, such as bacteria, fungi, and algae. Nanoparticles with antimicrobial properties, such as silver or copper, can be incorporated into coatings to inhibit the growth of these organisms, thereby protecting the artifact from biological decay. This is particularly useful for preserving organic materials like wood, leather, and textiles, which are especially susceptible to microbial degradation.

Table 7.1. Case studies: nanotechnology in preserving historical sites.

Historical Site	Location	Nanotechnology Used	Purpose	Outcome	Year	References
Colosseum	Rome, Italy	Nano-lime treatments	Consolidation of deteriorating stone surfaces	Improved structural integrity and long-term protection of limestone.	2016	[19]
Taj Mahal	Agra, India	Nano-coatings (silica-based)	Protecting marble surfaces from pollutants and weather	Significant reduction in surface discoloration and weathering effects.	2018	[20]
Cultural Heritage Sites in Florence	Florence, Italy	Calcium hydroxide nanoparticles	Consolidation of frescoes and plaster	Enhanced strength and reduced porosity of historical plaster and frescoes.	2017	[21]
Ancient Ruins of Pompeii	Pompeii, Italy	Nano-silica and nano-titanium dioxide coatings	Protection against environmental degradation	Reduced biological growth and surface deterioration.	2019	[22]
Church of Santa Maria Novella	Florence, Italy	Calcium hydroxide nanoparticles	Fresco preservation	Increased durability of frescoes with minimal aesthetic impact.	2015	[23]

RESTORATION OF ARTIFACTS USING NANOTECHNOLOGY

Nanotechnology has introduced highly precise and less invasive methods for cleaning and restoring artifacts, revolutionizing traditional restoration techniques. Cleaning delicate artifacts, such as ancient manuscripts, paintings, and sculptures, requires a gentle approach to avoid damaging the original materials [24]. Nanoparticles, due to their small size and controllable properties, offer a solution that allows for targeted cleaning. For example, nanomaterials like micelles or emulsions can be engineered to selectively remove dirt, grime, and previous restoration materials, such as old varnish, without harming the underlying artifact [25]. These nanomaterials work by encapsulating and breaking down contaminants at the molecular level, allowing them to be removed without the need for harsh chemicals or abrasive methods. This level of precision is especially important when dealing with fragile or irreplaceable objects, as it minimizes the risk of further deterioration. Additionally, nanotechnology enables restorers to clean artifacts in ways that were previously impossible, such as removing layers of pollution from outdoor sculptures or cleaning the delicate surfaces of ancient textiles without causing fiber damage [26].

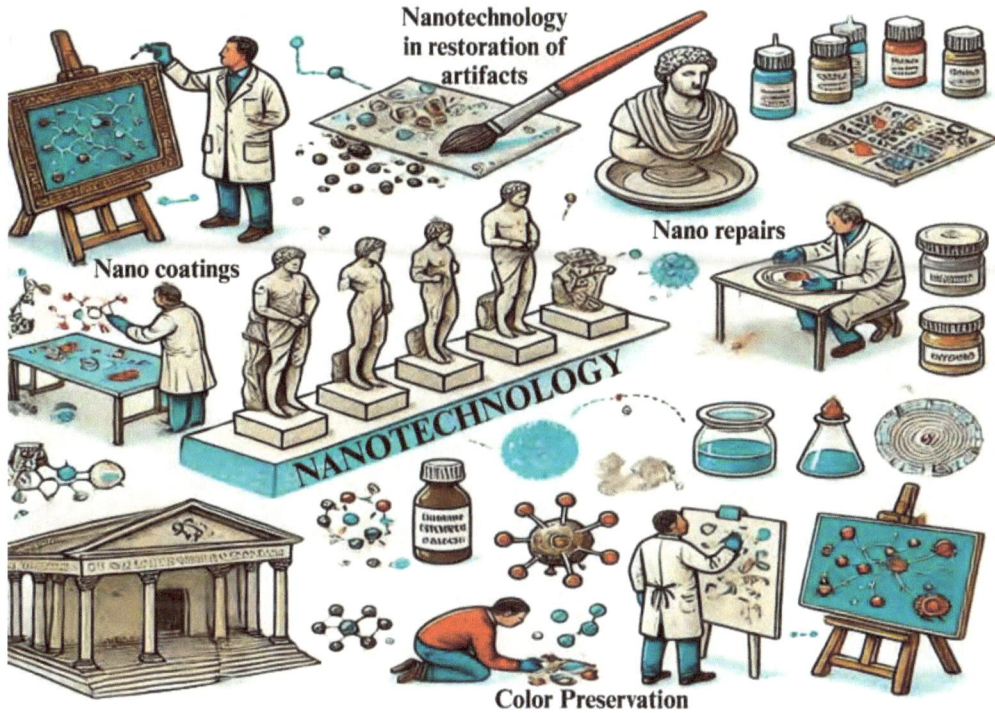

Fig. (7.1). Application of nanotechnology in preservation of artifacts.

Nanocomposites, which are materials that combine nanoparticles with traditional restoration materials, have become invaluable in the structural restoration of artifacts. These composites offer enhanced mechanical properties, such as increased strength, durability, and flexibility, which are essential for reinforcing damaged or deteriorating structures. For example, in the restoration of ancient frescoes or deteriorating stone sculptures, nanocomposites can be used to fill in cracks, stabilize the material, and prevent further decay [27]. Nanoparticles, such as calcium carbonate or silica, can be mixed with traditional binders to create a composite material that closely mimics the original structure of the artifact while providing additional strength. This approach ensures that the restoration is both effective and historically accurate, as the nanocomposites can be designed to match the physical and chemical properties of the original materials [28]. Due to their nanoscale dimensions, these particles can penetrate deep into the micro-cracks and voids of the artifact, reinforcing within. This internal strengthening helps to prevent further damage and ensures the longevity of the restored artifact.

Nanocomposites are also used in the restoration of metal artifacts, which are often subject to corrosion over time, as depicted in Fig. **7.2**. By incorporating nanoparticles into corrosion-resistant coatings or fillers, restorers can repair and protect metal objects, such as historical weapons, tools, or architectural elements, from further degradation [29]. The advantage of nanocomposites in this context is that they provide a protective layer that is both strong and thin, preserving the artifact's appearance while enhancing its structural integrity.

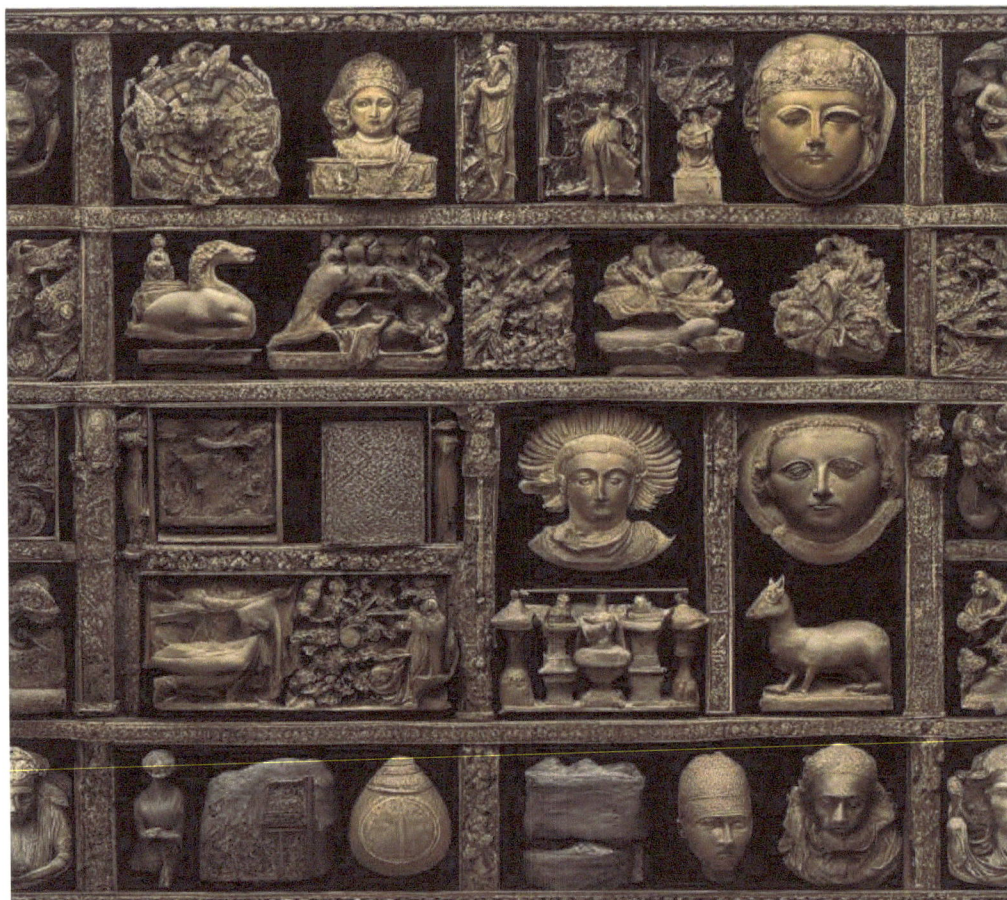

Fig. (7.2). Nanocomposites have played a significant role in the prevention of corrosion of sculptures and artifacts by incorporating nanoparticles into corrosion-resistant coatings or fillers.

Nanomaterials have also made significant advancements in the restoration of paintings and sculptures, two of the most challenging forms of art restoration due to their delicate nature and complex compositions, as highlighted in Table **7.2**. In painting restoration, nanoparticles are used to stabilize pigments and binders that have degraded over time. For example, nanoparticles of calcium hydroxide or barium hydroxide can be applied to paintings to neutralize acidic degradation products, which often cause the paint to crack or flake [30]. These nanoparticles interact with the damaged layers, restoring the pH balance and re-binding the pigments, which helps to preserve the color and integrity of the artwork. This method is particularly beneficial for frescoes and wall paintings, where traditional restoration methods may not reach deep into the porous layers. In the restoration of sculptures, nanomaterials can be employed to repair cracks, chips, and surface erosion while maintaining the original appearance of the piece [31]. For example, nanoscale silica or titanium dioxide can be used to fill in micro-cracks in marble or stone sculptures, providing a seamless repair that is invisible to the naked eye [32]. These nanoparticles bond with the original material, strengthening the structure without altering its texture or color. Additionally, nanomaterials can be used to protect restored sculptures from future damage. For example, a nano-coating can be applied to the surface of the sculpture to shield it from environmental factors such as pollution, moisture, and UV radiation, ensuring that the restoration lasts longer [33]. Nanotechnology has enabled restorers to recreate missing parts of sculptures with a level of precision that was previously unattainable. By using 3D printing technologies in combination with nanocomposites, it is possible to replicate intricate details and textures of the original sculpture, ensuring that the restoration is both aesthetically and structurally faithful to the original work [34]. This approach has been particularly useful in restoring fragmented statues or damaged architectural elements, where the missing pieces need to be recreated and integrated seamlessly into the existing structure.

Table 7.2. Case Studies: successful restoration projects using nanotechnology.

Artwork/Artifact	Location	Nanotechnology Used	Restoration Focus	Outcome	Year	References
Leonardo da Vinci's "The Last Supper"	Milan, Italy	Calcium hydroxide nanoparticles	Consolidation and surface cleaning.	Stabilized pigment and restored original color vibrancy.	2019	[35]
The Acropolis Sculptures	Athens, Greece	Nano-silica coatings	Cleaning and protection of marble surfaces.	Successful removal of pollutants and protection against further damage.	2017	[36]

(Table 7.2) cont.....

Artwork/Artifact	Location	Nanotechnology Used	Restoration Focus	Outcome	Year	References
Venetian Canvases (Tintoretto's Paintings)	Venice, Italy	Nano-emulsions for cleaning	Cleaning of aged varnish and restoration of original hues.	Restored clarity and color without damage to the original paint layers.	2018	[37]
Ancient Egyptian Statues	Cairo, Egypt	Nanocomposites for structural reinforcement	Repairing cracks and structural weaknesses.	Strengthened structure with minimal visual alteration.	2016	[38]
17th Century Frescoes in St. Ignatius Church	Rome, Italy	Calcium hydroxide and magnesium oxide nanoparticles	Surface consolidation and pigment stabilization.	Preserved vibrant colors and improved structural integrity.	-	[39]

NANOTECHNOLOGY IN NEW ARTISTIC MEDIUMS

Nanotechnology is not only revolutionizing traditional art forms but also opening up entirely new avenues for artistic expression. As an artistic medium, nanotechnology allows artists to manipulate materials at the molecular and atomic levels, creating works of art that were previously unimaginable [40]. This involves the use of nanomaterials like carbon nanotubes, quantum dots, and nanostructures to craft visual experiences that are dynamic, interactive, and often invisible to the naked eye [41]. These nanoscale materials can exhibit unique optical, electrical, and mechanical properties that enable the creation of art that changes with environmental conditions, such as light, temperature, or magnetic fields. For example, artists can design surfaces that shift colors or patterns based on the viewer's angle or proximity, creating a highly immersive and interactive experience [42]. The precision and control offered by nanotechnology allow for the creation of intricate and complex designs that challenge the traditional boundaries of art, merging science and creativity in unprecedented ways.

Nano-art is an emerging field where artists utilize nanotechnology as both a tool and a medium to create works of art on the nanoscale. This form of art often requires specialized equipment, such as scanning electron microscopes, to both create and view the artwork. Pioneering artists in this field, such as Cris Orfescu and Jonty Hurwitz, have pushed the boundaries of what is possible in art by using nanomaterials and techniques to create works that are not only visually stunning but also conceptually innovative [43]. For instance, Hurwitz is known for creating the world's smallest sculptures, which are so tiny they can fit within the eye of a needle and are only visible under a microscope [44]. These sculptures challenge our perceptions of scale and detail, pushing the limits of human craftsmanship and technological capability. Cris Orfescu, on the other hand, transforms scientific imagery from nanotechnology research into colorful and abstract pieces of art, blurring the line between science and aesthetics [45]. These artists are exploring the intersection of technology and creativity, using nanotechnology not just as a tool but as a means of expressing ideas about the microcosmic world and the hidden structures that govern our reality. Nano-art is, in essence, a fusion of science and art, where the beauty of the nanoscale world is revealed through the creative lens of the artist.

Nanomaterials are driving a wave of innovation in the art world, offering new possibilities for artistic creation that were previously out of reach, as illustrated in Fig. (**7.2**). The unique properties of nanomaterials—such as their ability to change color, conduct electricity, and exhibit extraordinary strength—have inspired artists to explore new techniques and forms of expression. For example, quantum dots, which are nanoscale semiconductor particles, can be used to create artworks that emit light in specific wavelengths, resulting in vibrant and dynamic color displays that are highly energy-efficient and long-lasting [46]. This has led to the development of artworks that glow in the dark, change colors under different lighting conditions, or even respond to the viewer's presence. Additionally, nanomaterials like graphene, known for their exceptional conductivity and flexibility, are being integrated into interactive installations where the artwork responds to touch or other stimuli, creating a more engaging experience for the audience. Nanomaterials are also being used to create environmentally conscious art. For example, artists are utilizing self-cleaning and air-purifying nano-coatings to develop pieces that not only captivate viewers but also contribute to environmental sustainability [47]. These artworks can actively break down pollutants in the air, turning art into a functional element in public spaces that promotes ecological well-being. Moreover, the strength and durability of nanomaterials allow for the creation of sculptures and installations that are both lightweight and resilient, enabling large-scale outdoor artworks that withstand harsh environmental conditions while maintaining their aesthetic appeal, depicted in Fig. (**7.3**). In addition to visual arts, nanotechnology is influencing other creative fields, such as fashion and textiles [48]. Designers are incorporating nanomaterials into fabrics to create clothing that changes color, repels stains, or even monitors the wearer's health. This blending of art, technology, and functionality represents a new frontier in creative expression, where aesthetics and practicality coexist seamlessly.

CHALLENGES AND ETHICAL CONSIDERATIONS

The application of nanotechnology in cultural heritage raises significant ethical questions, particularly regarding the preservation of authenticity and the potential for irreversible changes to valuable artifacts. One ethical dilemma centers on whether the use of nanomaterials, which can alter the original properties of artifacts, compromises the integrity of these cultural treasures. For example, introducing nano-coatings or nanocomposites to protect or restore an object might improve its durability, but it could also permanently alter its original material composition and appearance [49]. This raises concerns about the authenticity and originality of the artwork or artifact after intervention. Additionally, there is the question of consent, particularly in cases where artifacts belong to indigenous cultures or communities. The use of advanced technologies on culturally significant objects must be approached with sensitivity to the values and traditions of the communities to which they belong. Engaging these communities in decision-making processes and ensuring that interventions align with their cultural values is crucial for ethical preservation practices.

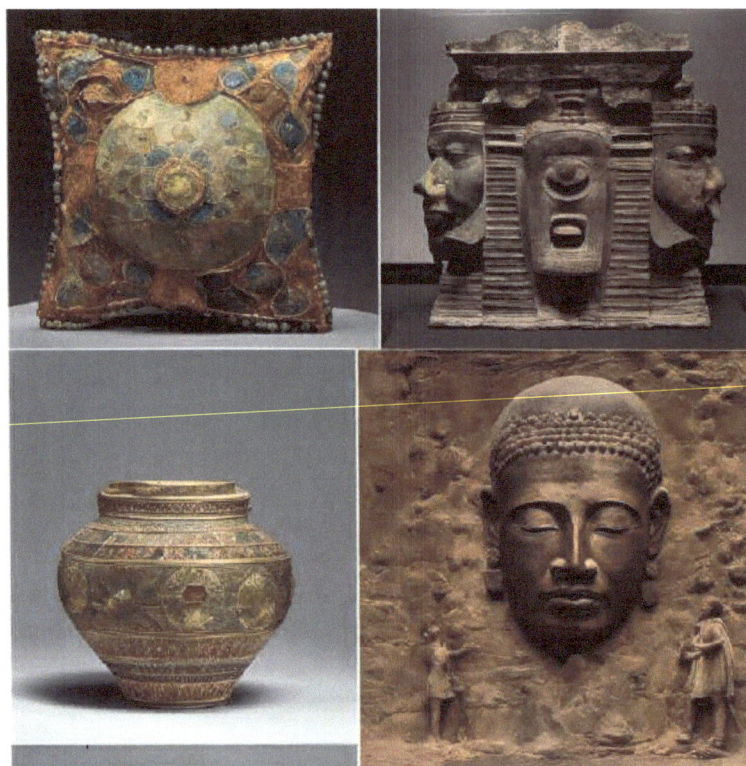

Fig. (7.3). Artistic paintings and sculptures made using nanoparticles remain durable for a longer period, withstanding the harsh environmental conditions.

Balancing tradition with innovation is a complex challenge in the context of nanotechnology in cultural heritage. While technological advancements offer new possibilities for preserving and restoring artifacts, there is often resistance from traditionalists who fear that these methods might overshadow or replace conventional techniques [50]. This tension between preserving time-honoured methods and embracing new technologies can create challenges in reaching consensus on the best approach to conservation. Traditional methods of restoration are rooted in historical practices that prioritize the use of materials and techniques similar to those originally employed by the artists or builders. Nanotechnology, by contrast, introduces modern materials and methods that may be foreign to these traditional practices [51]. The challenge lies in integrating these innovations without undermining the historical and cultural significance of the artifacts. It is essential to strike a balance where nanotechnology complements rather than replaces traditional restoration techniques, ensuring that cultural heritage is preserved in a way that respects its historical context while benefiting from modern advancements.

The potential risks and long-term effects of using nanotechnology in cultural heritage preservation and restoration are not fully understood, which presents a significant challenge. Nanomaterials, while effective in the short term, may have unforeseen consequences over time. For example, nano-coatings designed to protect surfaces from environmental damage might degrade or react with the underlying materials in unpredictable ways, potentially causing more harm than good in the long run. Additionally, the environmental impact of these nanomaterials must be considered, as the release of nanoparticles into the environment during the restoration process could pose ecological risks [52]. The long-term stability of nanomaterials used in restoration also raises concerns; while they may initially enhance the durability of artifacts, there is uncertainty about how they will age over decades or centuries. Continuous research and monitoring are required to assess the long-term effects of nanotechnology on restored artifacts, ensuring that these interventions do not lead to unintended deterioration or environmental harm. There is a need for regulatory frameworks that guide the safe and responsible use of nanotechnology in cultural heritage, balancing the potential benefits with the risks to ensure that preservation efforts do not inadvertently compromise the very artifacts they aim to protect [53].

FUTURE PERSPECTIVES

Nanotechnology is poised to play a transformative role in the future of art, giving rise to entirely new and innovative art forms that challenge our traditional understanding of creativity and expression. As artists continue to explore the potential of nanoscale materials and technologies, we can expect to see the emergence of art that is more interactive, immersive, and dynamic than ever before. For example, the use of quantum dots and other nanomaterials that change color, emit light, or react to environmental stimuli can lead to the creation of artworks that are not static but evolve, responding to changes in light, temperature, or even the viewer's presence. This opens up possibilities for art that is not just visually engaging but also emotionally and intellectually stimulating, as it interacts with its environment and audience in real time. Artists might create installations that change shape, texture, or color depending on the surrounding atmosphere, offering a new level of engagement and interactivity. The integration of nanotechnology with digital art forms could lead to the development of hybrid art experiences, where the physical and virtual worlds merge seamlessly. Augmented reality (AR) and virtual reality (VR) can be enhanced with nanomaterials that create more lifelike textures, making digital art feel more tangible. Imagine walking through a virtual gallery where you can not only see but also touch and feel the artworks, thanks to nanostructures that mimic the properties of real materials. This fusion of digital and nanotechnology-driven art forms has the potential to revolutionize how art is experienced, making it more accessible and engaging to a wider audience. Nanotechnology also holds promise for making art more sustainable and eco-friendly. Artists are increasingly exploring the use of nanomaterials that are biodegradable or have self-healing properties, reducing the environmental impact of their work. For example, nanotechnology could enable the creation of sculptures that repair themselves when damaged or installations that actively clean the air in their surroundings, blurring the line between art and functionality. This approach not only pushes the boundaries of creativity but also aligns with the growing global emphasis on sustainability and environmental consciousness in art and design. Looking forward, nanotechnology may also give rise to art forms that are entirely new and previously unimaginable. Artists may begin to work on the atomic level, creating structures and patterns that are invisible to the naked eye but can be revealed through specific conditions, such as light or magnification. This could lead to a new genre of "nano-art," where the artwork exists on a scale so small that it challenges our perceptions of size, space, and reality. The ability to manipulate materials at the nanoscale could result in art that integrates seamlessly with the human body, such as wearable art that changes appearance based on the wearer's emotions or health conditions. The future of nanotechnology in art is vast and filled with potential. As this technology continues to evolve, artists will likely explore new ways to integrate it into their work, creating art that is more dynamic, responsive, and aligned with the technological advancements of the 21st century. These emerging art forms will not only expand the possibilities of creative expression but also reshape how we perceive and interact with art in a world increasingly defined by innovation and technology.

CONCLUSION

The future of nanotechnology in art and cultural heritage holds immense promise, offering innovative solutions to the complex challenges of preservation, restoration, and artistic creation. As nanotechnology continues to advance, its applications in safeguarding cultural heritage will likely become more refined and widespread, enabling the protection of artifacts and monuments that were once considered beyond saving. Future developments may lead to even more precise and less invasive techniques, allowing conservators to preserve the authenticity of historical objects while enhancing their durability and resilience against environmental threats. Artists will have access to materials and tools that operate on a molecular level, allowing them to craft art that is dynamic, interactive, and responsive to the environment in ways that were previously unimaginable. This convergence of science and art has the potential to reshape both fields, leading to a future where technology and creativity are deeply intertwined.

In conclusion, the application of nanotechnology in art and cultural heritage is a powerful example of how innovation can serve as a bridge between the past and the future. Preservation and restoration efforts, traditionally constrained by the limitations of available materials and techniques, are being transformed by the precision and versatility of nanotechnology. This technology not only offers new methods for protecting and restoring valuable cultural artifacts but also respects the historical and cultural significance of these items by minimizing the impact of conservation interventions. However, the adoption of nanotechnology must be approached with careful consideration of the ethical implications and potential risks, ensuring that innovation does not come at the cost of authenticity or long-term preservation. As we move forward, it is essential to foster collaboration between scientists, conservators, and artists, creating a multidisciplinary approach that harnesses the full potential of nanotechnology while honouring the rich traditions of art and cultural heritage. Ultimately, the fusion of preservation, restoration, and innovation through nanotechnology will enable future generations to experience and appreciate the cultural treasures of the past in ways that are both meaningful and sustainable.

REFERENCES

[1]   Hulla, J.E.; Sahu, S.C.; Hayes, A.W. Nanotechnology. *Hum. Exp. Toxicol.,* **2015**, *34*(12), 1318-1321.
        [http://dx.doi.org/10.1177/0960327115603588] [PMID: 26614822]

[2]   Yilmaz, H.M.; Yakar, M.; Gulec, S.A.; Dulgerler, O.N. Importance of digital close-range photogrammetry in documentation of cultural heritage. *J. Cult. Herit.,* **2007**, *8*(4), 428-433.
        [http://dx.doi.org/10.1016/j.culher.2007.07.004]

[3]   Blanch, A.J.; Döblinger, M.; Rodríguez-Fernández, J. Simple and rapid high-yield synthesis and size sorting of multibranched hollow gold nanoparticles with highly tunable NIR plasmon resonances. *Small,* **2015**, *11*(35), 4550-4559.

[http://dx.doi.org/10.1002/smll.201500095] [PMID: 26068971]

[4]   Bardet, R.; Belgacem, N.; Bras, J. Flexibility and color monitoring of cellulose nanocrystal iridescent solid films using anionic or neutral polymers. *ACS Appl. Mater. Interfaces,* **2015**, *7*(7), 4010-4018.
        [http://dx.doi.org/10.1021/am506786t] [PMID: 25552332]

[5]   Goffredo, G.B.; Accoroni, S.; Totti, C.; Romagnoli, T.; Valentini, L.; Munafò, P. Titanium dioxide based nanotreatments to inhibit microalgal fouling on building stone surfaces. *Build. Environ.,* **2017**, *112*, 209-222.
        [http://dx.doi.org/10.1016/j.buildenv.2016.11.034]

[6]   Zhao, Z.; Khorasani, A.E.; Theodore, N.D.; Dhar, A.; Alford, T.L. Prediction of transmittance spectra for transparent composite electrodes with ultra-thin metal layers. *J. Appl. Phys.,* **2015**, *118*(20), 205304.
        [http://dx.doi.org/10.1063/1.4936316]

[7]   Verma, P.; Maheshwari, S.K. Applications of silver nanoparticles in diverse sectors. *Int. J. Nanodimens.,* **2019**, *10*(1), 18-36.

[8]   Wetzel, B.; Haupert, F.; Qiu Zhang, M. Epoxy nanocomposites with high mechanical and tribological performance. *Compos. Sci. Technol.,* **2003**, *63*(14), 2055-2067.
        [http://dx.doi.org/10.1016/S0266-3538(03)00115-5]

[9]   Smith, O.F. Object artifacts, image artifacts and conceptual artifacts: beyond the object into the event. *Artifact,* **2007**, *1*(1), 2-5.
        [http://dx.doi.org/10.1386/art.1.1.2_1]

[10]   Anderson, B.; Kearnes, M.; Doubleday, R. Geographies of nano-technoscience. *Area,* **2007**, *39*(2), 139-142.
        [http://dx.doi.org/10.1111/j.1475-4762.2007.00748.x]

[11]   Noel, V.A.A. New technologies in the preservation of cultural artifacts with spatial, temporal, corporeal, kinetic dimensions: artifacts in the trinidad carnival. *Studies in Digital Heritage,* **2017**, *1*(2), 251-268.
        [http://dx.doi.org/10.14434/sdh.v1i2.23277]

[12]   Akash, ; Harish, ; Chouhan, V.S.; Singhal, R.; Mukhopadhyay, A.K. Influence of nitrate on the growth of calcium hydroxide nanoparticles. *NanoWorld J.,* **2022**, *8*(S1).
        [http://dx.doi.org/10.17756/nwj.2022-s1-014]

[13]   Xu, C.; Qu, X. Cerium oxide nanoparticle: a remarkably versatile rare earth nanomaterial for biological applications. *NPG Asia Mater.,* **2014**, *6*(3), e90.
        [http://dx.doi.org/10.1038/am.2013.88]

[14]   Balandin, A.A. Thermal properties of graphene and nanostructured carbon materials. *Nat. Mater.,* **2011**, *10*(8), 569-581.
        [http://dx.doi.org/10.1038/nmat3064] [PMID: 21778997]

[15]   Decher, G. Fuzzy nanoassemblies: toward layered polymeric multicomposites. *Science,* **1997**, *277*(5330), 1232-1237.
        [http://dx.doi.org/10.1126/science.277.5330.1232]

[16]   Bhattacharya, K.; Davoren, M.; Boertz, J.; Schins, R.P.F.; Hoffmann, E.; Dopp, E. Titanium dioxide nanoparticles induce oxidative stress and DNA-adduct formation but not DNA-breakage in human lung cells. *Part. Fibre Toxicol.,* **2009**, *6*(1), 17.
        [http://dx.doi.org/10.1186/1743-8977-6-17] [PMID: 19545397]

[17]   Maan, A.M.C.; Hofman, A.H.; de Vos, W.M.; Kamperman, M. Recent developments and practical feasibility of polymer-based antifouling coatings. *Adv. Funct. Mater.,* **2020**, *30*(32), 2000936.
        [http://dx.doi.org/10.1002/adfm.202000936]

[18]   Lettieri, M.; Masieri, M.; Frigione, M. Durability to simulated bird guano of nano-filled oleo/hydrophobic coatings for the protection of stone materials. *Prog. Org. Coat.,* **2020**, *148*, 105900.

[http://dx.doi.org/10.1016/j.porgcoat.2020.105900]

[19]   Drdácký, M.; Slížková, Z.; Ziegenbalg, G. A Nano Approach to Consolidation of Degraded Historic Lime Mortars. *J. Nano Res.,* **2009,** *8,* 13-22.
[http://dx.doi.org/10.4028/www.scientific.net/JNanoR.8.13]

[20]   Bijapur, K.; Molahalli, V.; Shetty, A.; Toghan, A.; De Padova, P.; Hegde, G. Recent trends and progress in corrosion inhibitors and electrochemical evaluation. *Appl. Sci. (Basel),* **2023,** *13*(18), 10107.
[http://dx.doi.org/10.3390/app131810107]

[21]   Baglioni, P.; Carretti, E.; Chelazzi, D. Nanomaterials in art conservation. *Nat. Nanotechnol.,* **2015,** *10*(4), 287-290.
[http://dx.doi.org/10.1038/nnano.2015.38] [PMID: 25855252]

[22]   Chen, Y.; Wu, L.; Yao, W.; Wu, J.; Serdechnova, M.; Blawert, C.; Zheludkevich, M.L.; Yuan, Y.; Xie, Z.; Pan, F. "Smart" micro/nano container-based self-healing coatings on magnesium alloys: A review. *Journal of Magnesium and Alloys,* **2023,** *11*(7), 2230-2259.
[http://dx.doi.org/10.1016/j.jma.2023.06.006]

[23]   Baglioni, P.; Chelazzi, D.; Giorgi, R.; Poggi, G. Colloid and materials science for the conservation of cultural heritage: cleaning, consolidation, and deacidification. *Langmuir,* **2013,** *29*(17), 5110-5122.
[http://dx.doi.org/10.1021/la304456n] [PMID: 23432390]

[24]   Jackson, J.B.; Bowen, J.; Walker, G.; Labaune, J.; Mourou, G.; Menu, M.; Fukunaga, K. A survey of terahertz applications in cultural heritage conservation science. *IEEE Trans. Terahertz Sci. Technol.,* **2011,** *1*(1), 220-231.
[http://dx.doi.org/10.1109/TTHZ.2011.2159538]

[25]   Guerrero-Martínez, A.; Pérez-Juste, J.; Liz-Marzán, L.M. Recent progress on silica coating of nanoparticles and related nanomaterials. *Adv. Mater.,* **2010,** *22*(11), 1182-1195.
[http://dx.doi.org/10.1002/adma.200901263] [PMID: 20437506]

[26]   Gösele, U. How clean is too clean? *Nature,* **2006,** *440*(7080), 34-35.
[http://dx.doi.org/10.1038/440034a] [PMID: 16511478]

[27]   Masini, N.; Soldovieri, F. Integrated non-invasive sensing techniques and geophysical methods for the study and conservation of architectural, archaeological and artistic heritage. *J. Geophys. Eng.,* **2011,** *8*(3).
[http://dx.doi.org/10.1088/1742-2140/8/3/E01]

[28]   Kim, H.; Abdala, A.A.; Macosko, C.W. Graphene/polymer nanocomposites. *Macromolecules,* **2010,** *43*(16), 6515-6530.
[http://dx.doi.org/10.1021/ma100572e]

[29]   Camargo, P.H.C.; Satyanarayana, K.G.; Wypych, F. Nanocomposites: synthesis, structure, properties and new application opportunities. *Mater. Res.,* **2009,** *12*(1), 1-39.
[http://dx.doi.org/10.1590/S1516-14392009000100002]

[30]   Pandya, H.N.; Parikh, S.P.; Shah, M. Comprehensive review on application of various nanoparticles for the production of biodiesel. *Energy Sources A Recovery Util. Environ. Effects,* **2019,** 1-14.
[http://dx.doi.org/10.1080/15567036.2019.1648599]

[31]   Kakakhel, M.A.; Wu, F.; Gu, J.D.; Feng, H.; Shah, K.; Wang, W. Controlling biodeterioration of cultural heritage objects with biocides: A review. *Int. Biodeterior. Biodegradation,* **2019,** *143*, 104721.
[http://dx.doi.org/10.1016/j.ibiod.2019.104721]

[32]   Negi, G.S.; Anirbid, S.; Sivakumar, P. *Applications of silica and titanium dioxide nanoparticles in enhanced oil recovery: promises and challenges*; Petroleum Research, **2021.**
[http://dx.doi.org/10.1016/j.ptlrs.2021.03.001]

[33]   Taglietti, A. Introducing applied nano: an interdisciplinary open access journal showing how nanoscience can offer solutions to different problems and needs. *Appl. Nanosci.,* **2020,** *1*(1), 1-2.

[http://dx.doi.org/10.3390/applnano1010001]

[34]   Goyanes, A.; Det-Amornrat, U.; Wang, J.; Basit, A.W.; Gaisford, S. 3D scanning and 3D printing as innovative technologies for fabricating personalized topical drug delivery systems. *J. Control. Release,* **2016**, *234*, 41-48.
[http://dx.doi.org/10.1016/j.jconrel.2016.05.034] [PMID: 27189134]

[35]   Klimek, B. Application of colloidal calcium hydroxide nanoparticles for consolidation of damaged lime plaster in historical buildings. *Materialy Budowlane,* **2024**, *1*(10), 99-104.
[http://dx.doi.org/10.15199/33.2024.10.11]

[36]   Jones, R. The decoration and firing of ancient greek pottery: A review of recent investigations. *Advances in Archaeomaterials,* **2021**, *2*(2), 67-127.
[http://dx.doi.org/10.1016/j.aia.2021.07.002]

[37]   Chelazzi, D.; Bordes, R.; Giorgi, R.; Holmberg, K.; Baglioni, P. The use of surfactants in the cleaning of works of art. *Curr. Opin. Colloid Interface Sci.,* **2020**, *45*, 108-123.
[http://dx.doi.org/10.1016/j.cocis.2019.12.007]

[38]   Wegst, U.G.K.; Bai, H.; Saiz, E.; Tomsia, A.P.; Ritchie, R.O. Bioinspired structural materials. *Nat. Mater.,* **2015**, *14*(1), 23-36.
[http://dx.doi.org/10.1038/nmat4089] [PMID: 25344782]

[39]   Levy, E. Early modern jesuit arts and jesuit visual culture. *Journal of Jesuit Studies,* **2014**, *1*(1), 66-87.
[http://dx.doi.org/10.1163/22141332-00101005]

[40]   Dei, L.; Salvadori, B. Nanotechnology in cultural heritage conservation: nanometric slaked lime saves architectonic and artistic surfaces from decay. *J. Cult. Herit.,* **2006**, *7*(2), 110-115.
[http://dx.doi.org/10.1016/j.culher.2006.02.001]

[41]   Kessler, R. Engineered nanoparticles in consumer products: understanding a new ingredient. *Environ. Health Perspect.,* **2011**, *119*(3), a120-a125.
[http://dx.doi.org/10.1289/ehp.119-a120] [PMID: 21356630]

[42]   Yetisen, A.K.; Qu, H.; Manbachi, A.; Butt, H.; Dokmeci, M.R.; Hinestroza, J.P.; Skorobogatiy, M.; Khademhosseini, A.; Yun, S.H. Nanotechnology in Textiles. *ACS Nano,* **2016**, *10*(3), 3042-3068.
[http://dx.doi.org/10.1021/acsnano.5b08176] [PMID: 26918485]

[43]   Zukin, S. Gentrification: Culture and capital in the urban core. *Annu. Rev. Sociol.,* **1987**, *13*(1), 129-147.
[http://dx.doi.org/10.1146/annurev.so.13.080187.001021]

[44]   G. Colzani, C. Marconi, and F. Slavazzi, Greek and Roman Small Size Sculpture; De Gruyter, **2023**.
[http://dx.doi.org/10.1515/9783110741742]

[45]   Kang, J. Revealing the nanoscale world: digital recreation of nanofibre images. *International Journal of Arts and Technology,* **2013**, *6*(3), 286.
[http://dx.doi.org/10.1504/IJART.2013.055394]

[46]   Sperling, R.A.; Parak, W.J. Surface modification, functionalization and bioconjugation of colloidal inorganic nanoparticles. *Philos. Trans.- Royal Soc., Math. Phys. Eng. Sci.,* **2010**, *368*(1915), 1333-1383.
[http://dx.doi.org/10.1098/rsta.2009.0273] [PMID: 20156828]

[47]   Lee, D.; Koo, J.M.; Cho, Y.; Kim, J.; Kim, S.; Oh, D.X.; Jeon, H.; Park, J. Recent advances in utilizing surface-features of naturally derived nanocellulose and nanochitin for self-cleaning and purifying applications. *Bull. Korean Chem. Soc.,* **2024**, *45*(11), 880-895.
[http://dx.doi.org/10.1002/bkcs.12906]

[48]   Dhoundiyal, S.; Alam, M.A.; Kaur, A.; Maqsood, S.; Sharma, S.; Khan, S.A. *Biopolymers in sustainable textile dyeing and printing;* Springer Nature, **2024**, pp. 123-146.
[http://dx.doi.org/10.1007/978-981-97-0684-6_5]

[49] Caruso, F. Nanoengineering of Particle Surfaces. *Adv. Mater.,* **2001**, *13*(1), 11-22.
      [http://dx.doi.org/10.1002/1521-4095(200101)13:1<11::AID-ADMA11>3.0.CO;2-N]

[50] Freeman, C. The 'National System of Innovation' in historical perspective. *Camb. J. Econ.,* **1995**, *19*(1)
      [http://dx.doi.org/10.1093/oxfordjournals.cje.a035309]

[51] Alivisatos, P. The use of nanocrystals in biological detection. *Nat. Biotechnol.,* **2004**, *22*(1), 47-52.
      [http://dx.doi.org/10.1038/nbt927] [PMID: 14704706]

[52] Dhoundiyal, S.; Kaur, A.; Alam, M. A.; Sharma, A. the future of nanopesticides, nanoherbicides, and nanofertilizers. *CRC Press,* **2023**.
      [http://dx.doi.org/10.1201/9781003364429]

[53] I. Linkov; FK Satterstrom; Monica, J.; Hansen, S. F.; Davis, T. Nano risk governance: current developments and future perspectives *Nanotechnology Law & Business,* **2009**.

CHAPTER 8

Nanomaterials: Safety, Ethics, and Global Regulations

Abstract: Nanotechnology has rapidly emerged as a transformative force across various industries, but with this growth comes significant concerns about safety and regulation. This chapter explores the critical aspects of nanomaterial safety and regulation, starting with an introduction to the widespread use of nanomaterials in industry and research, highlighting the need for comprehensive safety measures. The discussion then shifts to the health and environmental risks associated with nanomaterials, including toxicity, exposure routes, and long-term effects, as well as their impact on ecosystems and wildlife. The chapter further examines the regulatory frameworks at both global and national levels, comparing approaches across different regions and outlining the challenges in regulating these materials, such as defining nanomaterials and assessing risks. Case studies of safety incidents are analyzed to illustrate real-world implications and lessons learned, from occupational exposure to product recalls. Finally, the chapter presents best practices for nanomaterial safety, emphasizing risk management strategies, the importance of sustainability, and the development of green nanotechnology to mitigate environmental impacts. This comprehensive overview provides a foundational understanding of the critical issues surrounding the safety and regulation of nanomaterials, emphasizing the need for continued vigilance and innovation in this rapidly evolving field.

Keywords: Case studies, Challenges, Environmental risks, Health risks, Regulatory frameworks, Regulation, Safety.

INTRODUCTION

Nanomaterials, due to their unique properties, have revolutionized various industries, including medicine, electronics, energy, and manufacturing. Their extremely small size and large surface area-to-volume ratio give them enhanced mechanical, electrical, and chemical properties compared to their bulk counterparts [1]. In industry and research, nanomaterials are utilized in applications ranging from drug delivery systems and cancer therapies to lightweight materials for aerospace and high-performance electronics. However, these same properties that make nanomaterials so valuable also pose potential risks to human health and the environment, making safety and regulation crucial [2]. Nanomaterials' small size allows them to interact with biological systems at the molecular and cellular levels, making them invaluable in fields like biotechnology and medicine. For example, nanoparticles can deliver drugs directly to cancer cells, reducing side effects and improving treatment efficacy. In the electronics industry, nanomaterials are used to develop faster and smaller transistors, enabling the creation of more powerful and compact devices. In energy, nanomaterials contribute to more efficient solar cells and batteries, potentially leading to sustainable energy solutions. Despite these advantages, the widespread use of nanomaterials in industry and research also raises concerns about their potential impact on health and the environment, necessitating stringent safety protocols and regulatory measures [3].

The rapid development and application of nanotechnology have outpaced the establishment of comprehensive safety regulations. The unique properties of nanomaterials, while beneficial in many applications, can also lead to unforeseen risks. For example, nanoparticles can easily penetrate biological barriers, such as the skin, lungs, or gastrointestinal tract, potentially causing toxicity or long-term health effects [4]. The small size of nanoparticles also means they can accumulate in the environment, posing risks to ecosystems. Moreover, the long-term impacts of exposure to nanomaterials are not yet fully understood, creating uncertainty around their safety. Given these potential risks, the regulation of nanomaterials is critical to ensuring their safe use. Regulatory frameworks must address the entire lifecycle of nanomaterials, from production and use to disposal. This includes establishing guidelines for exposure limits, toxicity testing, and environmental impact assessments. Additionally, regulation helps protect workers who handle nanomaterials in manufacturing and research settings, as well as consumers who use products containing nanomaterials [5]. Effective regulation also fosters public trust in nanotechnology, encouraging its adoption while mitigating potential risks. However, regulating nanomaterials presents significant challenges. Traditional regulatory approaches may not be suitable for nanomaterials due to their unique properties, requiring the development of new methods for risk assessment and safety evaluation. The lack of standardized definitions and measurement techniques for nanomaterials complicates regulatory efforts. Therefore, ongoing collaboration between industry, academia, and regulatory bodies is essential to develop robust safety standards and ensure that the benefits of nanotechnology are realized without compromising health or environmental safety [6].

HEALTH AND ENVIRONMENTAL RISKS OF NANOMATERIALS

The use of nanomaterials in various industries has raised concerns about their potential health and environmental risks. Due to their extremely small size and unique properties, nanoparticles can penetrate biological barriers, potentially causing toxicity in humans and animals. Inhalation, ingestion, or dermal exposure to certain nanomaterials may lead to respiratory issues, cellular damage, or inflammatory responses. Additionally, the environmental release of nanoparticles through industrial processes or consumer products poses risks to ecosystems. These particles can accumulate in soil and water, impacting microorganisms and entering the food chain. While nanotechnology holds immense promise, addressing these risks through rigorous research, regulation, and sustainable practices is crucial for its safe and responsible development, as depicted in Fig. (**8.1**).

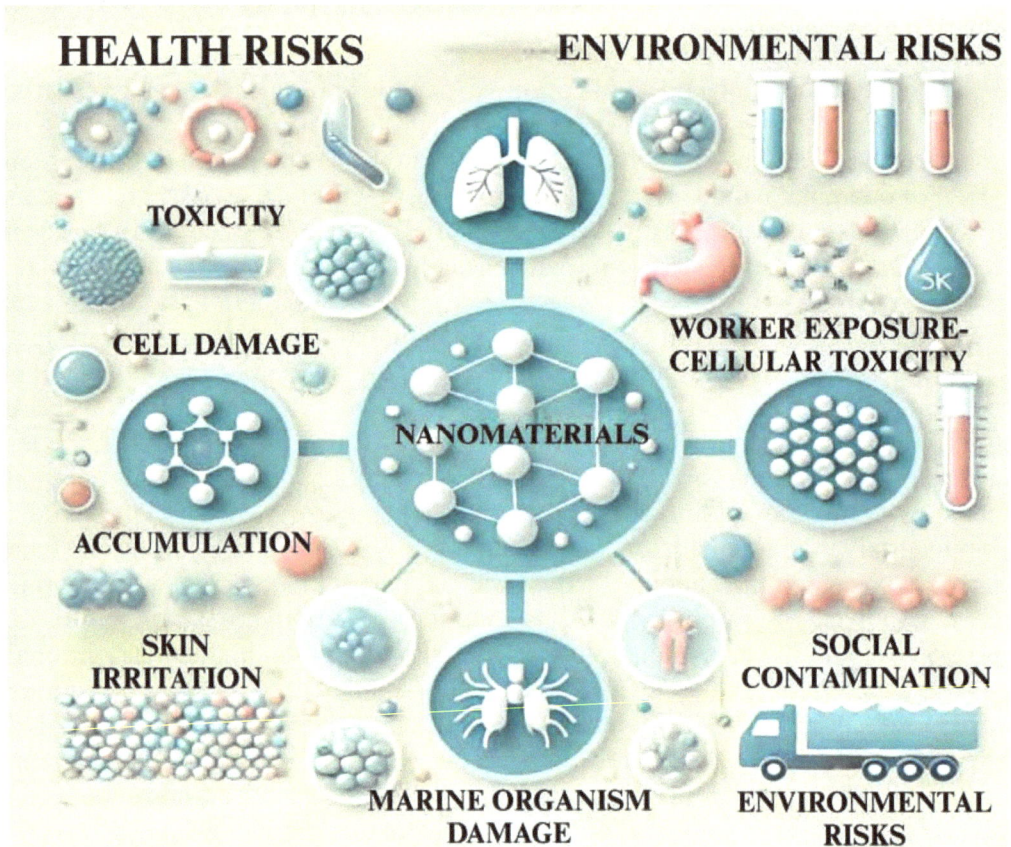

Fig. (8.1). Potential risks associated with the use of nanomaterials.

Health Risks

The rapid expansion of nanotechnology has raised concerns about the potential health risks associated with exposure to nanomaterials. Due to their small size and unique properties, nanoparticles can interact with biological systems in ways that are not fully understood, leading to potential toxicity and health hazards [7]. The toxicity of nanoparticles can vary depending on factors such as their size, shape, surface charge, and chemical composition, making it challenging to predict their effects on human health. These tiny particles can enter the body through various exposure routes, including inhalation, ingestion, and dermal contact, potentially causing harm to multiple organs and systems. The long-term health effects of nanoparticle exposure are still largely unknown, raising concerns about the potential for chronic health conditions that may not manifest until years after exposure [8]. Nanoparticles exhibit unique physicochemical properties that can contribute to their toxicity. For instance, their high surface area-to-volume ratio allows for increased chemical reactivity, which can lead to the generation of reactive oxygen species (ROS) [9]. These ROS can cause oxidative stress, inflammation, and damage to cellular components such as DNA, proteins, and lipids. Additionally, certain nanoparticles, like those made of heavy metals (*e.g.*, silver, cadmium), can release toxic ions that interfere with cellular functions [10]. The small size of nanoparticles also enables them to penetrate cell membranes and accumulate within cells, potentially disrupting normal cellular processes.

Toxicity studies have shown that nanoparticles can induce cytotoxicity, genotoxicity, and even apoptosis (programmed cell death), highlighting the importance of thoroughly assessing their safety before widespread use. Nanoparticles can enter the human body through several exposure routes, each posing distinct health risks. Inhalation is one of the most common exposure routes, particularly in occupational settings where nanoparticles are airborne [11]. When inhaled, nanoparticles can penetrate deep into the lungs, reaching the alveoli and potentially entering the bloodstream. This can lead to respiratory issues such as inflammation, fibrosis, and even lung cancer in extreme cases. Ingestion is another exposure route, which can occur unintentionally through contaminated food, water, or hand-to-mouth contact. Once ingested, nanoparticles can cross the gastrointestinal barrier and enter the circulatory system, potentially affecting organs such as the liver, kidneys, and intestines [12]. Dermal contact, while less commonly associated with severe toxicity, can still pose risks, particularly with nanoparticles that can penetrate the skin barrier. Once absorbed, these particles can enter the bloodstream and distribute throughout the body, raising concerns about systemic effects. The impact of nanoparticles on human organs and systems is a critical area of concern. In the respiratory system, inhaled nanoparticles can cause a range of issues, from mild irritation and inflammation to more severe conditions like chronic obstructive pulmonary disease (COPD) and lung cancer. Studies have shown that nanoparticles can trigger immune responses in the lungs, leading to chronic inflammation and scarring [13]. In the cardiovascular system, nanoparticles that enter the bloodstream can contribute to cardiovascular diseases by causing oxidative stress and inflammation in blood vessels, potentially leading to atherosclerosis, hypertension, and heart attacks.

Additionally, nanoparticles have been found to cross the blood-brain barrier, raising concerns about their impact on the nervous system. Neurotoxicity resulting from nanoparticle exposure can lead to cognitive impairments, neuroinflammation, and even neurodegenerative diseases like Alzheimer's and Parkinson's [14]. One of the most significant challenges in understanding the health risks of nanomaterials is the uncertainty surrounding their long-term effects. Many studies on nanoparticle toxicity have focused on short-term exposure, leaving gaps in knowledge about the chronic impacts of prolonged exposure. For instance, repeated or cumulative exposure to nanoparticles over time may lead to chronic health conditions, such as cancer, organ damage, or immune system dysfunction [15]. Some nanoparticles may persist in the body or accumulate in certain tissues, leading to delayed toxic effects that may not become apparent until years later. The unknown risks associated with nanomaterials also extend to vulnerable populations, such as children, pregnant women, and individuals with pre-existing health conditions, who may be more susceptible to the adverse effects of nanoparticles. As the use of nanomaterials continues to grow, it is essential to conduct long-term studies to fully understand their potential health risks and develop appropriate safety guidelines.

Environmental Risks

Nanomaterials, due to their novel properties and widespread use, present unique environmental risks that require careful consideration. These materials can persist and accumulate in the environment, potentially leading to harmful effects on soil, water, and air quality. The impact of nanomaterials on wildlife and ecosystems is also a growing concern, as they can disrupt ecological balance and threaten biodiversity. The ability of certain nanomaterials to bioaccumulate in organisms and biomagnify through the food chain raises significant concerns about their long-term environmental and health impacts [16]. Understanding these risks is crucial for developing effective strategies to mitigate the potential adverse effects of nanomaterials on the environment. One of the primary environmental concerns associated with nanomaterials is their persistence and accumulation in various ecosystems. Unlike conventional pollutants, nanomaterials can be highly resistant to degradation due to their stability and unique chemical properties. This persistence allows them to remain in the environment for extended periods, increasing the likelihood of accumulation in soil, water bodies, and sediments. For example, nanoparticles released from industrial processes, consumer products, or waste disposal can enter aquatic systems and settle in sediments, where they can persist for years [17]. This accumulation can lead to increased concentrations of nanomaterials in specific areas, potentially causing localized environmental harm. The persistence of nanomaterials also raises concerns about their long-term effects, as they may continue to interact with and potentially harm the environment long after their initial release. Nanomaterials can have significant effects on soil, water, and air quality, depending on their chemical composition and mode of entry into the environment. In soil, nanomaterials can alter microbial communities, disrupting essential processes like nutrient cycling and soil fertility. For instance, certain metal-based nanoparticles, such as silver and zinc oxide, have been shown to be toxic to soil microorganisms, reducing their populations and impairing soil health. In aquatic environments, nanomaterials can interfere with water quality by affecting the physical and chemical properties of water. For example, nanoparticles may increase water turbidity, reduce light penetration, and alter the availability of nutrients, affecting aquatic life. Moreover, nanomaterials can adsorb pollutants and transport them through water systems, potentially spreading contamination [18]. In the atmosphere, airborne nanoparticles can contribute to air pollution and pose inhalation risks to both humans and wildlife. These particles can also interact with atmospheric components, leading to the formation of secondary pollutants that further degrade air quality. The introduction of nanomaterials into the environment can have profound effects on wildlife and ecosystems. Nanomaterials can be toxic to a wide range of organisms, from microorganisms and plants to fish and mammals. For example, studies have shown that certain nanoparticles can inhibit the growth of algae, which form the base of many aquatic food webs [19]. The disruption of algal populations can have cascading effects on entire ecosystems, affecting the survival of fish and other aquatic species that rely on algae for food. In terrestrial ecosystems, nanomaterials can affect plant health by altering nutrient uptake and growth patterns. For instance, metal nanoparticles can accumulate in plant tissues, potentially reducing crop yields and affecting food security [20]. Nanomaterials can enter the bodies of animals through ingestion or inhalation, leading to toxic effects such as organ damage, reproductive issues, and even death. The impact of nanomaterials on wildlife and ecosystems underscores the need for comprehensive environmental assessments and protective measures. A significant environmental risk associated with nanomaterials is their potential for bioaccumulation and biomagnification. Bioaccumulation occurs when nanomaterials are absorbed by organisms at a rate faster than they can be excreted or metabolized, leading to an increase in concentration within the organism over time. This process can be particularly concerning for species at the lower levels of the food chain, such as plankton and small fish, which may accumulate nanomaterials from their environment. Biomagnification, on the other hand, refers to the increasing concentration of nanomaterials as they move up the food chain. Predatory species, including humans, may be exposed to higher levels of nanomaterials due to their consumption of contaminated prey [21]. For example, if nanoparticles accumulate in small fish, larger fish that eat them may have even higher concentrations of these materials in their bodies. This process can have serious implications for the health of top predators and raise concerns about the safety of consuming contaminated seafood. The potential for bioaccumulation and biomagnification of nanomaterials highlights the importance of monitoring and regulating their release into the environment.

REGULATORY FRAMEWORKS FOR NANOMATERIALS

Various regulatory bodies around the world continuously monitor the safety and efficacy of the nanomaterials. Some case studies highlighting the regulation of such nanomaterials are depicted in Table **8.1**.

Table 8.1. Case studies of regulation of nanomaterials.

Case Study	Country/Region	Nanomaterial	Regulatory Body	Regulation/Guideline	Outcome	References
REACH Regulation	European Union	Various nanomaterials	European Chemicals Agency (ECHA)	The REACH regulation was extended to include nanomaterials, requiring specific data on nanomaterial properties and risks for registration.	The inclusion of nanomaterials in REACH led to greater transparency in the EU market, with companies required to provide detailed information on nanomaterials, including toxicity, environmental impact, and exposure data. This regulation set a precedent for nano-specific legislation globally.	[22]

(Table 8.1) cont.....

Case Study	Country/Region	Nanomaterial	Regulatory Body	Regulation/Guideline	Outcome	References
FDA Guidelines for Nanotechnology in Products	USA	Nanomaterials in food, cosmetics, drugs	Food and Drug Administration (FDA)	FDA issued guidelines for the use of nanomaterials in various products, emphasizing the need for safety testing, risk assessment, and proper labeling of nanomaterials in consumer products.	Companies using nanomaterials in their products were required to submit safety data to the FDA, ensuring consumer safety. The guidelines prompted more rigorous testing and assessment of nano-enabled products, particularly in sensitive industries like food and cosmetics.	[23]
Australia's National Industrial Chemicals Notification and Assessment Scheme (NICNAS)	Australia	Engineered nanomaterials	National Industrial Chemicals Notification and Assessment Scheme (NICNAS)	NICNAS included engineered nanomaterials under its assessment, requiring manufacturers and importers to notify the agency before introducing nanomaterials into the market.	Australia strengthened its regulatory oversight on nanomaterials, leading to improved monitoring and assessment of nanomaterials in commercial products. This helped in ensuring the safe use of nanomaterials and addressed public concerns related to potential risks.	[24]

(Table 8.1) cont.....

Case Study	Country/Region	Nanomaterial	Regulatory Body	Regulation/Guideline	Outcome	References
Canada's Environmental Protection Act (CEPA) Amendments	Canada	Nanomaterials in the environment	Environment and Climate Change Canada (ECCC)	Amendments to CEPA mandated that nanomaterials undergo a thorough environmental assessment before being released into the environment. The amendment also emphasized the need for pollution prevention.	The amendments led to stricter control over the use of nanomaterials in industrial applications, especially those with potential environmental impact. The focus on pollution prevention pushed companies to adopt safer and more sustainable practices when dealing with nanomaterials.	[25]
China's Draft Regulation on Nanomaterials	China	Various nanomaterials	Ministry of Ecology and Environment (MEE)	Draft regulation requiring mandatory safety assessments, environmental impact studies, and proper labeling for nanomaterials, especially in consumer and industrial products.	Though still in the draft phase, the regulation signaled China's intent to tighten controls on nanomaterials. The focus on safety and environmental impact aligned with international trends, and companies began adjusting their practices in anticipation of stricter regulations.	[26]

Global Regulatory Landscape for Nanomaterials

The global regulatory landscape for nanomaterials is complex and continually evolving, as countries and international organizations strive to balance the technological benefits of nanotechnology with the need to ensure safety and environmental protection. International standards, such as those developed by the International Organization for Standardization (ISO) and the Organisation for Economic Co-operation and Development (OECD), play a critical role in guiding the safe use of nanomaterials across borders [27]. These organizations provide frameworks for the testing, characterization, and risk assessment of nanomaterials, helping to harmonize regulatory approaches globally. However, the regulatory landscape varies significantly across regions, with different countries adopting unique approaches based on their priorities and regulatory cultures. In Europe, the European Union (EU) has implemented stringent regulations through the REACH (Registration, Evaluation, Authorisation, and Restriction of Chemicals) framework, which requires comprehensive safety data and risk assessments for nanomaterials [28]. The EU also mandates specific labeling requirements for products containing nanomaterials, ensuring transparency for consumers. In the United States, regulatory oversight is more fragmented, with various agencies such as the Environmental Protection Agency (EPA) and the Food and Drug Administration (FDA) responsible for different aspects of nanomaterial regulation [29]. The U.S. approach tends to be more flexible, focusing on case-by-case evaluations and relying on existing chemical safety laws to address nanomaterial risks. In Asia, regulatory approaches vary widely, with countries like Japan and South Korea developing advanced nanomaterial regulations, while others, such as China and India, are still in the process of establishing comprehensive frameworks [30]. Japan has been a leader in promoting voluntary industry standards and has focused on research to better understand the risks associated with nanomaterials. Meanwhile, China, as a major producer of nanomaterials, is increasingly recognizing the need for stronger regulations and has begun to implement more rigorous safety assessments. These varying approaches reflect the diverse economic, industrial, and environmental contexts of different regions, underscoring the importance of international cooperation and harmonization in the regulation of nanomaterials. International organizations like ISO and OECD are pivotal in establishing global standards for nanomaterials [31]. ISO develops technical standards that guide the safe production, handling, and disposal of nanomaterials, providing a common language for industries and regulators worldwide. These standards address issues such as the characterization of nanomaterials, measurement techniques, and safety testing protocols, ensuring that nanomaterials are evaluated consistently across different jurisdictions. The OECD, on the other hand, focuses on promoting responsible development and use of nanotechnology through its Working Party on

Manufactured Nanomaterials (WPMN). The OECD develops guidelines for the safety testing of nanomaterials, focusing on their potential impacts on health and the environment [32]. These guidelines help ensure that nanomaterials are thoroughly assessed before they enter the market, reducing the risk of harmful effects.

The regulatory approaches to nanomaterials vary across different regions, reflecting diverse priorities and regulatory frameworks. In Europe, the REACH regulation is one of the most comprehensive frameworks for nanomaterial regulation. Under REACH, companies must provide detailed information on the properties and potential risks of nanomaterials, including their toxicological and environmental effects [33]. The EU also requires that products containing nanomaterials be labelled, allowing consumers to make informed choices. Additionally, the European Chemicals Agency (ECHA) plays a central role in assessing the safety of nanomaterials and ensuring compliance with REACH requirements. In the United States, nanomaterial regulation is less centralized, with different agencies overseeing various aspects of nanomaterial safety [34]. The EPA regulates nanomaterials under the Toxic Substances Control Act (TSCA), focusing on their environmental impacts, while the FDA oversees the safety of nanomaterials in food, cosmetics, and pharmaceuticals. The U.S. regulatory approach tends to be more flexible, allowing for case-by-case evaluations of nanomaterials rather than imposing blanket regulations [35]. This approach is intended to encourage innovation while ensuring that potential risks are adequately addressed. In Asia, regulatory approaches to nanomaterials vary widely. Japan has been at the forefront of nanomaterial regulation, promoting voluntary industry standards and investing in research to better understand the risks associated with nanotechnology. South Korea has also developed advanced regulatory frameworks, with a focus on ensuring the safety of nanomaterials in consumer products. In contrast, China, as one of the world's largest producers of nanomaterials, has been slower to establish comprehensive regulations but is increasingly recognizing the need for stronger oversight [36]. China has recently implemented more rigorous safety assessments for nanomaterials, particularly in the context of occupational exposure and environmental protection. India, while still in the early stages of nanomaterial regulation, is also beginning to develop guidelines and safety standards to address the growing use of nanotechnology.

National Regulations and Guidelines

National regulations and guidelines for nanomaterials vary widely across major countries, reflecting different regulatory priorities, industrial contexts, and public health concerns. The European Union (EU), the United States (US), and other key countries have developed specific frameworks to manage the risks associated with nanomaterials, each with its unique approach. The EU's REACH (Registration, Evaluation, Authorisation, and Restriction of Chemicals) regulation is one of the most stringent and comprehensive frameworks globally, requiring detailed safety data, risk assessments, and registration for any chemical substance produced or imported in significant quantities, including nanomaterials [37]. REACH aims to protect human health and the environment by ensuring that all nanomaterials on the EU market are thoroughly evaluated for potential risks, with specific provisions for labeling and consumer transparency. In contrast, the United States takes a more fragmented approach, with various agencies such as the Environmental Protection Agency (EPA) and the Food and Drug Administration (FDA) responsible for different aspects of nanomaterial regulation. The EPA regulates nanomaterials primarily under the Toxic Substances Control Act (TSCA), focusing on environmental impacts and requiring manufacturers to submit pre-manufacture notifications for new nanomaterials [38]. Meanwhile, the FDA oversees the safety of nanomaterials in food, drugs, and cosmetics, applying existing regulatory frameworks to assess the safety of products containing nanomaterials on a case-by-case basis.

Other countries like Japan, China, and Australia have also developed their regulatory approaches, each with varying levels of stringency and focus. Japan, known for its advanced technology sector, emphasizes voluntary guidelines and industry-led initiatives, promoting the safe development and use of nanomaterials through collaboration between government, industry, and academia [39]. China's regulatory approach is evolving rapidly, reflecting its status as a leading producer of nanomaterials. The country has begun to implement stricter safety assessments and controls, particularly in industries where nanomaterial exposure is common, such as manufacturing and consumer products. Australia, meanwhile, has integrated nanomaterial safety into its broader chemical regulatory framework, requiring manufacturers to provide detailed information on the properties and potential risks of nanomaterials before they can be marketed [40]. In the European Union, REACH is the cornerstone of nanomaterial regulation. This framework mandates that companies provide comprehensive data on the safety and environmental impact of nanomaterials, including detailed toxicological and ecotoxicological information. REACH also requires that any product containing nanomaterials be clearly labelled, ensuring transparency for consumers. The European Chemicals Agency (ECHA) plays a central role in evaluating the safety of nanomaterials and enforcing compliance with REACH requirements. By placing the burden of proof on manufacturers, REACH aims to ensure that only safe nanomaterials are available on the European market.

In the United States, the regulatory landscape for nanomaterials is more decentralized, with the EPA and FDA playing key roles. The EPA regulates nanomaterials under TSCA, requiring manufacturers to submit pre-manufacture notifications for new nanomaterials and conduct risk assessments. The EPA also has the authority to restrict or ban nanomaterials that pose significant risks to human health or the environment [41]. The FDA, meanwhile, applies existing regulatory frameworks to evaluate the safety of nanomaterials in food, drugs, and cosmetics. This case-by-case approach allows the FDA to assess the safety of nanomaterials in specific products, taking into account their unique properties and potential risks. In Japan, the government has adopted a more collaborative approach to nanomaterial regulation, emphasizing voluntary guidelines and industry-led initiatives. The Japanese government works closely with industry and academia to develop best practices for the safe handling and use of nanomaterials. This approach reflects Japan's commitment to promoting innovation while ensuring that nanomaterials are used safely and responsibly. China, as a major producer of nanomaterials, has recognized the need for stronger regulations and has begun to implement more rigorous safety assessments [42]. Chinese regulations now require companies to conduct comprehensive risk assessments for nanomaterials, particularly in industries where exposure is common. This shift towards stricter regulation reflects China's growing awareness of the potential risks associated with nanomaterials and its commitment to protecting public health and the environment.

Australia integrates nanomaterial safety into its broader chemical regulatory framework. The National Industrial Chemicals Notification and Assessment Scheme (NICNAS) requires manufacturers to provide detailed information on the properties and risks of nanomaterials. This information is used to assess the safety of nanomaterials before they can be marketed in Australia, ensuring that only safe nanomaterials are available to consumers [43]. The differences in regulatory approaches across countries highlight the varying priorities and strategies in managing nanomaterial risks. The EU's precautionary approach, exemplified by REACH, emphasizes comprehensive safety assessments and consumer transparency, placing a strong emphasis on protecting public health and the environment. In contrast, the US adopts a more flexible, case-by-case approach, relying on existing chemical safety laws and focusing on innovation and market access. Japan's approach is characterized by industry collaboration and voluntary guidelines, reflecting its emphasis on technological advancement and responsible innovation [44]. China's evolving regulatory landscape demonstrates a growing commitment to stricter controls and safety assessments, driven by its status as a leading producer of nanomaterials. Australia, like the EU, integrates nanomaterial safety into its broader chemical regulation framework, ensuring that detailed risk assessments are conducted before nanomaterials can be marketed. These differences in regulatory approaches underscore the importance of international collaboration and harmonization to address the global nature of nanomaterial production and use. As nanotechnology continues to advance, the development of consistent and effective regulations across countries will be crucial to ensuring the safe and sustainable use of nanomaterials worldwide.

Challenges in Nanomaterial Regulation

Regulating nanomaterials presents a unique set of challenges, largely due to the distinct properties of these materials and the rapid pace of technological advancement, as illustrated in Fig. (**8.2**). One of the fundamental challenges lies in defining nanomaterials themselves, as their size, shape, and composition can vary significantly, making it difficult to create a standardized regulatory framework. Nanomaterials are typically defined as materials with at least one dimension smaller than 100 nanometers, but this definition does not fully capture the complexity of their behavior at the nanoscale. The shape of nanoparticles—whether spherical, tubular, or irregular—can significantly influence their properties and interactions with biological systems, complicating the regulatory process [45]. Additionally, nanomaterials can be composed of a wide range of substances, from metals and oxides to carbon-based materials, each with different potential risks. Establishing a clear and universally accepted definition of nanomaterials is therefore a critical challenge that regulators face. Another significant challenge is the development of appropriate testing and risk assessment protocols for nanomaterials. Traditional testing methods used for bulk materials may not be adequate for assessing the safety of nanomaterials, as their small size and unique properties can result in different toxicological profiles [46]. For example, nanoparticles may penetrate biological barriers more easily, accumulate in specific organs, or exhibit increased reactivity compared to larger particles of the same substance. As a result, new testing protocols that consider the specific behaviors and effects of nanomaterials are needed. This includes assessing potential exposure routes, such as inhalation, ingestion, and dermal contact, as well as evaluating the potential impacts on human health and the environment [47]. However, developing these protocols is a complex and time-consuming process, requiring significant research and validation before they can be implemented in regulatory frameworks.

The lack of long-term data on the effects of nanomaterials further complicates risk assessment and regulation. Since nanotechnology is a relatively new field, there is limited information on the long-term health and environmental impacts of nanomaterials. This uncertainty makes it difficult for regulators to predict the potential risks associated with nanomaterials, particularly for chronic exposure scenarios. For instance, while some studies have shown that certain nanoparticles can cause toxicity in cells or animals, the long-term effects on human health, such as cancer or respiratory diseases, are still largely unknown [48]. Similarly, the long-term environmental fate of nanomaterials, including their persistence, accumulation, and potential to bio-magnify through food chains, remains poorly understood. This lack of data creates uncertainty in regulatory decision-making, often leading to conservative approaches that may hinder innovation and the development of new nanotechnologies. The rapid pace of nanotechnology innovation poses a significant challenge for regulators. As new nanomaterials and applications are developed, regulatory frameworks must adapt quickly to address emerging risks. However, the regulatory process is often slower than the pace of technological advancement, leading to gaps in oversight and potential safety concerns [49]. This issue is particularly pronounced in industries like cosmetics, electronics, and medicine, where the commercialization of new nanomaterials often outpaces the development of corresponding safety regulations.

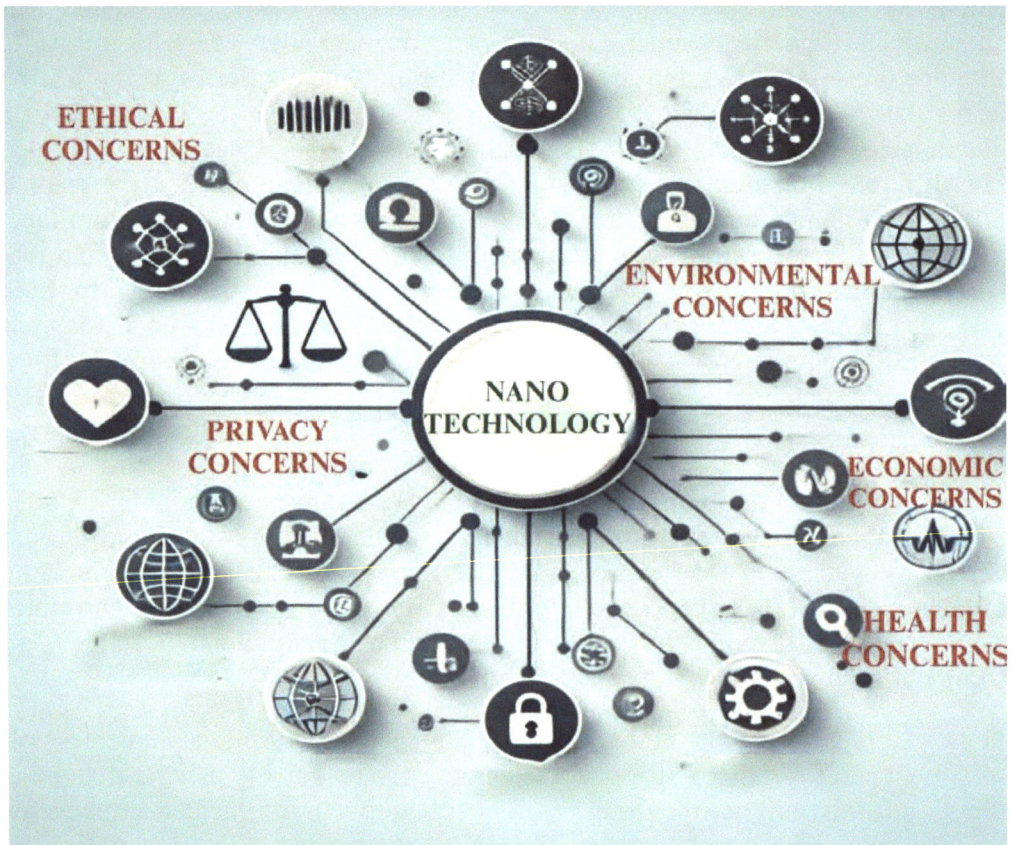

Fig. (8.2). Concerns with the use of nanomaterials.

CASE STUDIES ON SAFETY INCIDENTS INVOLVING NANOMATERIALS

Case studies on safety incidents involving nanomaterials highlight the real-world challenges and risks associated with their use, particularly in occupational settings, the environment, and consumer products, as listed in Table **8.2**. Occupational exposure and accidents involving nanomaterials have raised significant concerns about worker safety. For instance, workers in industries such as manufacturing, electronics, and cosmetics are often exposed to nanoparticles during production processes, which can lead to health issues such as respiratory problems, skin irritation, and, in some cases, long-term diseases like lung fibrosis [50]. A notable example is the exposure of workers to carbon nanotubes, which are similar in shape and size to asbestos fibers, raising concerns about their potential to cause similar health effects, such as mesothelioma. These incidents have underscored the importance of proper safety protocols, including the use of personal protective equipment (PPE), ventilation systems, and regular health monitoring of workers. Lessons learned from these cases emphasize the need for strict enforcement of safety standards, ongoing worker training, and the development of industry-specific guidelines to mitigate risks. In addition to workplace incidents, environmental contamination from nanomaterials has emerged as a critical issue [51]. Case studies have documented incidents where nanomaterials have been released into the environment, leading to contamination of soil, water, and air. For example, silver nanoparticles, commonly used in antimicrobial coatings, have been found to leach into water bodies, where they can accumulate and disrupt aquatic ecosystems. The impact of such contamination can be profound, affecting not only wildlife but also human health through the food chain. Cleanup efforts in these cases have often been challenging due to the persistence and mobility of nanoparticles in the environment [52]. These incidents have prompted a reevaluation of waste management practices and highlighted the need for more stringent environmental regulations to prevent nanomaterial pollution. Product recalls and public safety concerns have also brought attention to the potential risks of nanomaterials in consumer products. Several high-profile recalls have involved products containing nanomaterials that were found to pose safety risks. For instance, sunscreen products containing nano-sized titanium dioxide and zinc oxide have raised concerns about skin penetration and potential toxicity, leading to recalls and increased scrutiny from regulatory agencies [53]. In another case, a series of dietary supplements containing nano silver were recalled due to safety concerns over their potential to cause argyria, a condition that turns the skin blue-gray due to silver accumulation. These incidents have led to greater consumer awareness and demand for transparency in product labeling, as well as more proactive regulatory actions to protect public safety. Regulatory bodies such as the U.S. Food and Drug Administration (FDA) and the European

Medicines Agency (EMA) have responded by tightening regulations on nanomaterials in consumer products, requiring more rigorous safety testing and clearer labeling to ensure that consumers are informed about the presence of nanomaterials in the products they use.

Table 8.2. Case studies on safety incidents involving nanomaterials.

Incident	Location	Nanomaterial Involved	Industry/Application	Description of Incident	Consequences/Outcome	References
Explosion in a metal nanoparticle manufacturing plant	China	Metal nanoparticles	Manufacturing	A dust explosion occurred in a plant producing metal nanoparticles due to improper handling and storage of nanopowders, leading to the ignition of the material.	The incident led to multiple fatalities and injuries. As a consequence, stricter safety protocols were enforced across the industry, including better ventilation, dust management, and worker training. This case highlighted the need for robust safety measures in nanoparticle manufacturing environments and contributed to global awareness regarding the hazards of handling nanomaterials in powder form.	[54]
Consumer exposure to silver nanoparticles in antibacterial clothing	USA	Silver nanoparticles	Consumer products (textiles)	Consumers reported skin irritation after wearing clothing treated with silver nanoparticles for antibacterial properties. Concerns arose over nanoparticle release during washing.	The incident led to increased scrutiny of nano-enhanced consumer products, prompting regulatory bodies like the FDA and EPA to investigate the safety of silver nanoparticles. Subsequent studies showed potential environmental impact due to nanoparticle release into wastewater. As a result, manufacturers were encouraged to conduct more thorough safety assessments and provide clear labeling of nano-enabled products.	[55]

(Table 8.2) cont.....

Incident	Location	Nanomaterial Involved	Industry/Application	Description of Incident	Consequences/Outcome	References
Nanotube exposure in research laboratories	USA	Carbon nanotubes	Academic research	Several researchers experienced respiratory issues after being exposed to airborne carbon nanotubes in poorly ventilated laboratories.	The incident led to the implementation of stricter safety protocols in laboratories working with nanomaterials. Protective equipment, improved ventilation, and better training for handling nanomaterials were mandated. Additionally, this incident influenced guidelines by organizations like NIOSH, raising awareness about the potential health risks associated with prolonged exposure to certain nanomaterials.	[56]
Environmental spill of nanomaterials in river	Brazil	Titanium dioxide nanoparticles	Chemical industry	A spill of titanium dioxide nanoparticles from a chemical plant contaminated a nearby river, leading to concerns about the impact on aquatic life and water quality.	The incident caused public outcry and led to fines for the company responsible. Environmental agencies conducted extensive testing, which revealed potential harm to aquatic organisms. In response, stricter regulations for containment and disposal of nanomaterials in the chemical industry were implemented. This case emphasized the need for robust environmental safeguards when dealing with nanomaterials, particularly in proximity to sensitive ecosystems.	[57]

(Table 8.2) cont.....

Incident	Location	Nanomaterial Involved	Industry/Application	Description of Incident	Consequences/Outcome	References
Worker health concerns in nanoparticle coating facility	France	Nanoparticles used in coatings	Manufacturing	Workers in a nanoparticle coating facility reported respiratory problems and skin irritation after prolonged exposure to nanoparticle aerosols, leading to concerns about occupational safety.	The facility was temporarily shut down for a comprehensive safety review. The incident prompted the introduction of better protective measures for workers, including enhanced ventilation, protective clothing, and regular health monitoring. It also led to a broader discussion on the need for industry-wide standards to protect workers from potential health risks associated with nanomaterials.	[58]

Legal Cases and Liability Issues

The emergence of nanotechnology has brought about complex legal cases and liability issues related to nanomaterial exposure and potential damage. Litigation involving nanomaterials typically arises from claims of harm due to exposure in occupational settings, consumer products, or environmental contamination. One of the first significant legal cases involved a group of workers exposed to nanoparticles in a manufacturing plant, who developed serious respiratory illnesses [59]. These workers filed lawsuits against the manufacturer, claiming that the company failed to provide adequate protective measures and did not disclose the potential risks associated with nanomaterial exposure. Such cases highlight the legal responsibility of employers to ensure the safety of their workers when handling nanomaterials, which can include implementing safety protocols, providing proper protective equipment, and conducting regular health monitoring. These lawsuits often revolve around proving causation—establishing a direct link between nanomaterial exposure and the harm suffered—which can be challenging due to the limited long-term data on nanomaterial toxicity.

In addition to occupational exposure, legal cases have emerged from consumers who have been harmed by products containing nanomaterials. For example, there have been lawsuits involving cosmetics and skincare products that contain nanoparticles, with consumers alleging skin irritation, allergic reactions, or other health issues. In some instances, these cases have led to product recalls and significant financial settlements [60]. The legal implications for manufacturers in such cases are profound, as they may face liability for failing to conduct thorough safety testing, inadequately labeling products, or not warning consumers of potential risks. These cases have underscored the need for manufacturers to rigorously assess the safety of nanomaterials before incorporating them into products, as well as to ensure transparency with consumers through clear labeling and warnings. Environmental litigation is another area where nanomaterial liability issues arise. Companies responsible for the release of nanomaterials into the environment—whether through industrial processes, waste disposal, or product degradation—can face lawsuits from communities or environmental groups [61]. These cases often involve claims of environmental damage, such as contamination of water sources or harm to local ecosystems, and may result in costly clean-up efforts and legal penalties. The difficulty in tracing environmental contamination back to a specific source, combined with the challenges in assessing long-term environmental impacts, can complicate these legal battles. Nonetheless, these cases highlight the importance of environmental stewardship and adherence to regulations governing the disposal and handling of nanomaterials. The implications of these legal cases extend beyond the courtroom, influencing both manufacturers and regulators. For manufacturers, the risk of litigation serves as a powerful incentive to adopt safer practices, conduct thorough risk assessments, and ensure compliance with existing regulations [62]. Companies that fail to do so not only risk financial losses but also damage to their reputation and consumer trust. For regulators, legal cases involving nanomaterials often act as a catalyst for stricter regulations and oversight. High-profile lawsuits can expose gaps in current regulatory frameworks, prompting authorities to revise guidelines, enforce stricter safety standards, and enhance monitoring of nanomaterial use in various industries.

BEST PRACTICES FOR NANOMATERIAL SAFETY

Effectively managing the risks associated with nanomaterials requires a comprehensive approach that incorporates safe design and synthesis of nanomaterials, engineering controls, personal protective equipment (PPE), and continuous monitoring of health and environmental impacts. Safe design and synthesis begin with understanding the intrinsic properties of nanomaterials, such as size, shape, surface chemistry, and reactivity, and tailoring these properties to minimize potential hazards [63]. For example, modifying the surface of nanoparticles to reduce their toxicity or engineering them to degrade harmlessly after use can significantly reduce risks. This proactive approach, often referred to as "safety by design," emphasizes the importance of integrating safety considerations early in the development process rather than addressing risks after materials have been manufactured and commercialized [64]. Engineering controls are another critical component of risk management, particularly in occupational settings where workers may be exposed to nanomaterials during production, handling, or disposal. These controls include ventilation systems, fume hoods, and containment strategies that prevent the release of nanoparticles into the workplace environment. Engineering controls are often coupled with personal protective equipment (PPE), such as gloves, masks, and protective clothing, designed to shield workers from direct exposure to nanomaterials. Proper training on the use of PPE and adherence to safety protocols are essential to ensure that these protective measures are effective. By combining engineering controls with PPE, workplaces can significantly reduce the risk of exposure and potential health impacts associated with nanomaterials [65]. Monitoring and surveillance play a vital role in managing the long-term risks of nanomaterials. Continuous monitoring of both health and environmental impacts is necessary to detect early signs of harm and to respond swiftly. This includes regular health checks for workers exposed to nanomaterials, as well as environmental monitoring to track the presence of nanomaterials in air, water, and soil. Advanced detection techniques, such as real-time sensors and analytical tools, can provide valuable data on exposure levels and potential risks. Surveillance programs also contribute to building a knowledge base of the long-term effects of nanomaterials, which is currently limited due to the relatively recent introduction of these materials [66]. Effective monitoring helps ensure that any emerging risks are identified and addressed promptly, thereby protecting both human health and the environment.

As the field of nanotechnology continues to expand, there is a growing emphasis on sustainability and green nanotechnology to mitigate the environmental impact of nanomaterials and processes. Developing environmentally friendly nanomaterials involves designing materials that are non-toxic, biodegradable, and capable of being recycled or safely disposed of at the end of their lifecycle. Green nanotechnology prioritizes the use of renewable resources, reducing the reliance on hazardous chemicals, and minimizing waste during production. For example, researchers are exploring the use of natural polymers and plant-based materials to create sustainable nanocomposites that maintain functionality without posing environmental risks [67]. This shift towards greener materials is driven by both regulatory pressures and consumer demand for eco-friendly products. Reducing the environmental footprint of nanotechnology also requires rethinking production processes to make them more energy-efficient and less resource-intensive. This includes adopting cleaner production techniques that reduce emissions, waste, and water use, as well as exploring alternative energy sources, such as solar or wind power, to drive manufacturing processes. By improving the efficiency of nanomaterial synthesis and reducing resource consumption, companies can lower their environmental impact while maintaining the economic viability of their operations. Furthermore, implementing life cycle assessments (LCAs) helps quantify the environmental impact of nanomaterials from cradle to grave, guiding decision-making towards more sustainable practices [68]. Green nanotechnology is not only about minimizing harm but also about maximizing the positive contributions of nanomaterials to sustainability, such as in renewable energy, water purification, and pollution control technologies.

FUTURE DIRECTIONS

As the field of nanotechnology rapidly evolves, future directions in nanomaterial regulation will be shaped by emerging trends and technological advances that demand more sophisticated and adaptable regulatory frameworks. Anticipated changes in global regulations are likely to involve the harmonization of standards across different countries and regions to address the international nature of nanomaterial production, trade, and usage. As nanotechnology applications become increasingly global, regulatory bodies such as the International Organization for Standardization (ISO) and the Organisation for Economic Co-operation and Development (OECD) are expected to play a pivotal role in establishing uniform guidelines that ensure consistency in safety assessments, labeling, and risk management practices [69]. This could lead to the development of international regulatory frameworks that streamline the approval process for nanomaterials, reduce trade barriers, and enhance collaboration between regulatory agencies worldwide. Another anticipated change is the shift toward more proactive regulation that addresses potential risks early in the development cycle. Traditionally, regulations have often followed technological innovations, reacting to risks after they have been identified. However, with nanomaterials, there is a growing recognition of the need for precautionary regulation—a more forward-looking approach that anticipates and mitigates risks before they become significant. This could involve tighter scrutiny during the research and development phase, requiring companies to conduct comprehensive safety evaluations before nanomaterials are commercialized. Additionally, regulators may introduce more stringent post-market surveillance requirements to monitor the long-term impacts of nanomaterials and adjust regulations as new data becomes available.

Technological advances in nanomaterial synthesis, characterization, and application are also expected to significantly impact future regulations. As new nanomaterials with novel properties are developed, existing regulatory frameworks may need to be updated to accommodate these innovations. For example, the advent of self-assembling nanomaterials, nanoscale 3D printing, and advanced nanocomposites will likely require regulators to revise definitions, testing protocols, and safety guidelines to account for these materials' unique behaviors and interactions with biological systems and the environment [70]. The rise of nanomedicine and personalized nanotechnology—where nanomaterials are tailored for specific medical applications—also presents new regulatory challenges. Ensuring the safety and efficacy of these highly specialized nanomaterials will require a more nuanced approach to regulation, potentially involving more collaboration between regulatory agencies, medical professionals, and researchers. This could lead to the development of regulatory pathways that are specifically designed for nanomedicine, balancing the need for innovation with patient safety.

CONCLUSION

The chapter on nanomaterial safety and regulation underscores the importance of implementing robust safety measures and regulatory frameworks in response to the growing use of nanotechnology across various sectors. It is clear that while nanomaterials offer immense potential, their unique properties also pose significant health and environmental risks that require careful management. The analysis of global and national regulatory approaches reveals a need for harmonized standards and more precise definitions to address the complexities of nanomaterial regulation.

Through case studies on safety incidents, the chapter highlights the real-world consequences of inadequate safety measures and the importance of proactive risk management. The exploration of best practices demonstrates that sustainable and green nanotechnology approaches are crucial for reducing the environmental footprint of nanomaterials and ensuring their safe use. The chapter then emphasizes the need for continued innovation in regulatory frameworks and safety practices, as well as the importance of ongoing research to better understand the long-term impacts of nanomaterials. This chapter advocates for a balanced approach that fosters technological advancement while prioritizing human health and environmental protection.

REFERENCES

[1]   Hood, E. Nanotechnology: looking as we leap. *Environ. Health Perspect.,* **2004,** *112*(13), A740-A749.
       [http://dx.doi.org/10.1289/ehp.112-a740] [PMID: 15345364]

[2]   Charitidis, C.A.; Georgiou, P.; Koklioti, M.A.; Trompeta, A.F.; Markakis, V. Manufacturing
       nanomaterials: from research to industry. *Manuf. Rev. (Les Ulis),* **2014,** *1*, 11.
       [http://dx.doi.org/10.1051/mfreview/2014009]

[3]   Tayeb, A.; Mahmoud, M.; Geddawy, H. Enhancing solar still productivity: Use of nanomaterials.
       International Journal of Industry and Sustainable Development, **2023,** *4*(1), 81-89.
       [http://dx.doi.org/10.21608/ijisd.2023.319713]

[4]   Aravamudhan, S. Do Engineered Nanoparticles Penetrate into Cells? *J. Nanomed. Nanotechnol.,* **2013,**
       4(5).
       [http://dx.doi.org/10.4172/2157-7439.1000e132]

[5]   Duncan, T.V. Applications of nanotechnology in food packaging and food safety: Barrier materials,
       antimicrobials and sensors. *J. Colloid Interface Sci.,* **2011,** *363*(1), 1-24.
       [http://dx.doi.org/10.1016/j.jcis.2011.07.017] [PMID: 21824625]

[6]   Oberdörster, G.; Maynard, A.; Donaldson, K.; Castranova, V.; Fitzpatrick, J.; Ausman, K.; Carter, J.; Karn, B.; Kreyling, W.; Lai, D.; Olin, S.; Monteiro-Riviere, N.; Warheit, D.; Yang, H. Principles for characterizing the potential human health effects from exposure to nanomaterials: elements of a screening strategy. *Part. Fibre Toxicol.,* **2005**, *2*(1), 8.
[http://dx.doi.org/10.1186/1743-8977-2-8] [PMID: 16209704]

[7]   Kim, J.; Piao, Y.; Hyeon, T. Multifunctional nanostructured materials for multimodal imaging, and simultaneous imaging and therapy. *Chem. Soc. Rev.,* **2009**, *38*(2), 372-390.
[http://dx.doi.org/10.1039/B709883A] [PMID: 19169455]

[8]   Connor, E.E.; Mwamuka, J.; Gole, A.; Murphy, C.J.; Wyatt, M.D. Gold nanoparticles are taken up by human cells but do not cause acute cytotoxicity. *Small,* **2005**, *1*(3), 325-327.
[http://dx.doi.org/10.1002/smll.200400093] [PMID: 17193451]

[9]   Dhoundiyal, S.; Alam, M.A. Overcoming the Limitations of Therapeutic Strategies to Combat Pancreatic Cancer using Nanotechnology. *Curr. Cancer Drug Targets,* **2023**, *23*(9), 697-717.
[http://dx.doi.org/10.2174/1568009623666230329085618] [PMID: 36999420]

[10]   Chen, F.; Cai, W. Nanomedicine for targeted photothermal cancer therapy: where are we now? *Nanomedicine (Lond.),* **2015**, *10*(1), 1-3.
[http://dx.doi.org/10.2217/nnm.14.186] [PMID: 25597770]

[11]   Na, H.B.; Lee, J.H.; An, K.; Park, Y.I.; Park, M.; Lee, I.S.; Nam, D.H.; Kim, S.T.; Kim, S.H.; Kim, S.W.; Lim, K.H.; Kim, K.S.; Kim, S.O.; Hyeon, T. Development of a T1 contrast agent for magnetic resonance imaging using MnO nanoparticles. *Angew. Chem. Int. Ed.,* **2007**, *46*(28), 5397-5401.
[http://dx.doi.org/10.1002/anie.200604775] [PMID: 17357103]

[12]   Mitchell, M.J.; Billingsley, M.M.; Haley, R.M.; Wechsler, M.E.; Peppas, N.A.; Langer, R. Engineering precision nanoparticles for drug delivery. *Nat. Rev. Drug Discov.,* **2021**, *20*(2), 101-124.
[http://dx.doi.org/10.1038/s41573-020-0090-8] [PMID: 33277608]

[13]   Oberdörster, G.; Sharp, Z.; Atudorei, V.; Elder, A.; Gelein, R.; Kreyling, W.; Cox, C. Translocation of inhaled ultrafine particles to the brain. *Inhal. Toxicol.,* **2004**, *16*(6-7), 437-445.
[http://dx.doi.org/10.1080/08958370490439597] [PMID: 15204759]

[14]   Kessler, R. Engineered nanoparticles in consumer products: understanding a new ingredient. *Environ. Health Perspect.,* **2011**, *119*(3), a120-a125.
[http://dx.doi.org/10.1289/ehp.119-a120] [PMID: 21356630]

[15]   Senapati, S.; Mahanta, A.K.; Kumar, S.; Maiti, P. Controlled drug delivery vehicles for cancer treatment and their performance. *Signal Transduct. Target. Ther.,* **2018**, *3*(1), 7.
[http://dx.doi.org/10.1038/s41392-017-0004-3] [PMID: 29560283]

[16]   Nel, A.E.; Mädler, L.; Velegol, D.; Xia, T.; Hoek, E.M.V.; Somasundaran, P.; Klaessig, F.; Castranova, V.; Thompson, M. Understanding biophysicochemical interactions at the nano–bio interface. *Nat. Mater.,* **2009**, *8*(7), 543-557.
[http://dx.doi.org/10.1038/nmat2442] [PMID: 19525947]

[17]   Islam, N.; Osama Eljamal. A mini-review on transportation and fate of silver released from consumer products: Ecological risk assessments. *Proc. Int. Exch. Innov. Conf. Eng. Sci. IEICES,* **2022**, *8*, 52-61.
[http://dx.doi.org/10.5109/5909062]

[18]   Giraldo, J.P.; Landry, M.P.; Faltermeier, S.M.; McNicholas, T.P.; Iverson, N.M.; Boghossian, A.A.; Reuel, N.F.; Hilmer, A.J.; Sen, F.; Brew, J.A.; Strano, M.S. Plant nanobionics approach to augment photosynthesis and biochemical sensing. *Nat. Mater.,* **2014**, *13*(4), 400-408.
[http://dx.doi.org/10.1038/nmat3890] [PMID: 24633343]

[19]   Khan, I.; Saeed, K.; Khan, I. Nanoparticles: Properties, applications and toxicities. *Arab. J. Chem.,* **2019**, *12*(7), 908-931.
[http://dx.doi.org/10.1016/j.arabjc.2017.05.011]

[20]   Zulfiqar, F.; Ashraf, M. Nanoparticles potentially mediate salt stress tolerance in plants. *Plant Physiol.*

Biochem., **2021**, *160*, 257-268.
[http://dx.doi.org/10.1016/j.plaphy.2021.01.028] [PMID: 33529801]

[21]   Relyea, R.A. New effects of Roundup on amphibians: Predators reduce herbicide mortality; herbicides induce antipredator morphology. *Ecol. Appl.,* **2012**, *22*(2), 634-647.
[http://dx.doi.org/10.1890/11-0189.1] [PMID: 22611860]

[22]   Kemmlein, S.; Herzke, D.; Law, R.J. Brominated flame retardants in the European chemicals policy of REACH—Regulation and determination in materials. *J. Chromatogr. A,* **2009**, *1216*(3), 320-333.
[http://dx.doi.org/10.1016/j.chroma.2008.05.085] [PMID: 18582893]

[23]   Tyner, K.M.; Zou, P.; Yang, X.; Zhang, H.; Cruz, C.N.; Lee, S.L. Product quality for nanomaterials: current U.S. experience and perspective. *Wiley Interdisc. Rev. Nanomed. Nanobiotechnol.,* **2015**, *7*(5), 640-654.
[http://dx.doi.org/10.1002/wnan.1338] [PMID: 25641690]

[24]   Cushen, M.; Kerry, J.; Morris, M.; Cruz-Romero, M.; Cummins, E. Nanotechnologies in the food industry – Recent developments, risks and regulation. *Trends Food Sci. Technol.,* **2012**, *24*(1), 30-46.
[http://dx.doi.org/10.1016/j.tifs.2011.10.006]

[25]   Marmot, M.; Friel, S.; Bell, R.; Houweling, T.A.J.; Taylor, S. Closing the gap in a generation: health equity through action on the social determinants of health. *Lancet,* **2008**, *372*(9650), 1661-1669.
[http://dx.doi.org/10.1016/S0140-6736(08)61690-6] [PMID: 18994664]

[26]   Chaudhry, Q.; Castle, L. Food applications of nanotechnologies: An overview of opportunities and challenges for developing countries. *Trends Food Sci. Technol.,* **2011**, *22*(11), 595-603.
[http://dx.doi.org/10.1016/j.tifs.2011.01.001]

[27]   Moher, D.; Liberati, A.; Tetzlaff, J.; Altman, D.G. *Preferred Reporting Items for Systematic Reviews and Meta-Analyses: The PRISMA Statement*; PubMed, **2009**.

[28]   The European Union summary report on trends and sources of zoonoses, zoonotic agents and food-borne outbreaks in 2017. *EFSA J.,* **2018**, *16*(12), e05500.
[http://dx.doi.org/10.2903/j.efsa.2018.5500] [PMID: 32625785]

[29]   Schwartz, L.M.; Woloshin, S. Medical Marketing in the United States, 1997-2016. *JAMA,* **2019**, *321*(1), 80-96.
[http://dx.doi.org/10.1001/jama.2018.19320] [PMID: 30620375]

[30]   Tay, A.K.; Carlsson, J. Psychosocial treatment outcomes of common mental disorders vary widely in persons in low- and middle-income countries affected by humanitarian crises and refugees in high-income countries. *BJPsych Open,* **2022**, *8*(4), e100.
[http://dx.doi.org/10.1192/bjo.2022.73] [PMID: 35642349]

[31]   Miljkovic, D. International organizations and arrangements: Pivotal countries and manipulations. *Econ. Model.,* **2009**, *26*(6), 1398-1402.
[http://dx.doi.org/10.1016/j.econmod.2009.07.010]

[32]   Rasmussen, K.; Rauscher, H.; Kearns, P.; González, M.; Riego Sintes, J. Developing OECD test guidelines for regulatory testing of nanomaterials to ensure mutual acceptance of test data. *Regul. Toxicol. Pharmacol.,* **2019**, *104*, 74-83.
[http://dx.doi.org/10.1016/j.yrtph.2019.02.008] [PMID: 30831158]

[33]   Schwirn, K.; Voelker, D.; Galert, W.; Quik, J.; Tietjen, L. Environmental Risk Assessment of Nanomaterials in the Light of New Obligations Under the REACH Regulation: Which Challenges Remain and How to Approach Them? *Integr. Environ. Assess. Manag.,* **2020**, *16*(5), 706-717.
[http://dx.doi.org/10.1002/ieam.4267] [PMID: 32175661]

[34]   Pepic, I.; Hafner, A.; Lovric, J.; Perina Lakos, G. Nanotherapeutics in the EU: an overview on current state and future directions. *Int. J. Nanomedicine,* **2014**, *9*, 1005-1023.
[http://dx.doi.org/10.2147/IJN.S55359] [PMID: 24600222]

[35]   Hristovski, K.; Westerhoff, P.; Crittenden, J. An approach for evaluating nanomaterials for use as

packed bed adsorber media: A case study of arsenate removal by titanate nanofibers. *J. Hazard. Mater.,* **2008**, *156*(1-3), 604-611.
[http://dx.doi.org/10.1016/j.jhazmat.2007.12.073] [PMID: 18242828]

[36]   Tian, G.; Gu, Z.; Zhou, L.; Yin, W.; Liu, X.; Yan, L.; Jin, S.; Ren, W.; Xing, G.; Li, S.; Zhao, Y. Mn^{2+} dopant-controlled synthesis of NaYF$_4$:Yb/Er upconversion nanoparticles for *in vivo* imaging and drug delivery. *Adv. Mater.,* **2012**, *24*(9), 1226-1231.
[http://dx.doi.org/10.1002/adma.201104741] [PMID: 22282270]

[37]   Katharina Stahl, A. The Impact of China's Rise on the EU's Geopolitical Reach and Interests in Africa. *Eur. Foreign Aff. Rev.,* **2011**, *16*(4), 427-446.
[http://dx.doi.org/10.54648/EERR2011030]

[38]   Nel, A.E.; Mädler, L.; Velegol, D.; Xia, T.; Hoek, E.M.V.; Somasundaran, P.; Klaessig, F.; Castranova, V.; Thompson, M. Understanding biophysicochemical interactions at the nano–bio interface. *Nat. Mater.,* **2009**, *8*(7), 543-557.
[http://dx.doi.org/10.1038/nmat2442] [PMID: 19525947]

[39]   Tsuda, H. Risk assessment studies of nanomaterials in Japan and other countries. *PubMed,* **2010**, *11*(1), 13-14.
[PMID: 20593919]

[40]   Benke, G.; Dennekamp, M.; Priestly, B.; Sim, M. Engineered nanomaterials: Feasibility of establishing exposure standards and using control banding in Australia, **2010**.

[41]   Britt Erickson. EPA Moves to Ban Uses of Trichloroethylene. *C&EN Global Enterprise,* **2016**, *94*(49), 20-20.
[http://dx.doi.org/10.1021/cen-09449-notw13]

[42]   Silvestre, C.; Duraccio, D.; Cimmino, S. Food packaging based on polymer nanomaterials. *Prog. Polym. Sci.,* **2011**, *36*(12), 1766-1782.
[http://dx.doi.org/10.1016/j.progpolymsci.2011.02.003]

[43]   UNS, D. O. C. Lectures and Workshop: In Series of Nanotechnology and Nanomaterial Plasma Science and Technology for Nanomaterial Engineering. *Proceeding of Chemistry Conferences,* **2017**, *2*(1).
[http://dx.doi.org/10.20961/pcc.v2i1.15052]

[44]   Katao, K. Nanomaterials may call for a reconsideration of the present Japanese chemical regulatory system. *Clean Technol. Environ. Policy,* **2006**, *8*(4), 251-259.
[http://dx.doi.org/10.1007/s10098-006-0060-9]

[45]   Buzea, C.; Pacheco, I.I.; Robbie, K. Nanomaterials and nanoparticles: Sources and toxicity. *Biointerphases,* **2007**, *2*(4), MR17-MR71.
[http://dx.doi.org/10.1116/1.2815690] [PMID: 20419892]

[46]   Klaine, S.J.; Koelmans, A.A.; Horne, N.; Carley, S.; Handy, R.D.; Kapustka, L.; Nowack, B.; von der Kammer, F. Paradigms to assess the environmental impact of manufactured nanomaterials. *Environ. Toxicol. Chem.,* **2012**, *31*(1), 3-14.
[http://dx.doi.org/10.1002/etc.733] [PMID: 22162122]

[47]   Handy, R.D.; Cornelis, G.; Fernandes, T.; Tsyusko, O.; Decho, A.; Sabo-Attwood, T.; Metcalfe, C.; Steevens, J.A.; Klaine, S.J.; Koelmans, A.A.; Horne, N. Ecotoxicity test methods for engineered nanomaterials: Practical experiences and recommendations from the bench. *Environ. Toxicol. Chem.,* **2012**, *31*(1), 15-31.
[http://dx.doi.org/10.1002/etc.706] [PMID: 22002667]

[48]   Lee, J.S.; Han, M.S.; Mirkin, C.A. Colorimetric detection of mercuric ion (Hg^{2+}) in aqueous media using DNA-functionalized gold nanoparticles. *Angew. Chem. Int. Ed.,* **2007**, *46*(22), 4093-4096.
[http://dx.doi.org/10.1002/anie.200700269] [PMID: 17461429]

[49]   Huang, X.; Zhang, W.; Guan, G.; Song, G.; Zou, R.; Hu, J. Design and functionalization of the NIR-

responsive photothermal semiconductor nanomaterials for cancer theranostics. *Acc. Chem. Res.,* **2017**, *50*(10), 2529-2538.
[http://dx.doi.org/10.1021/acs.accounts.7b00294] [PMID: 28972736]

[50] Dhoundiyal, S.; Alam, M.A.; Kaur, A.; Sharma, S. Nanomedicines: Impactful Approaches for Targeting Pulmonary Diseases. *Pharm. Nanotechnol.,* **2024**, *12*(1), 14-31.
[http://dx.doi.org/10.2174/2211738511666230525151106] [PMID: 37231722]

[51] Dixit, R.; Wasiullah, ; Malaviya, D.; Pandiyan, K.; Singh, U.; Sahu, A.; Shukla, R.; Singh, B.; Rai, J.; Sharma, P.; Lade, H.; Paul, D. Bioremediation of Heavy Metals from Soil and Aquatic Environment: An Overview of Principles and Criteria of Fundamental Processes. *Sustainability (Basel),* **2015**, *7*(2), 2189-2212.
[http://dx.doi.org/10.3390/su7022189]

[52] Dhoundiyal, S.; Kaur, A.; Alam, M.A.; Sharma, A. *The Future of Nanopesticides, Nanoherbicides, and Nanofertilizers*; CRC Press, **2023**.
[http://dx.doi.org/10.1201/9781003364429-7]

[53] Kockler, J.; Oelgemöller, M.; Robertson, S.; Glass, B. Influence of Titanium Dioxide Particle Size on the Photostability of the Chemical UV-Filters Butyl Methoxy Dibenzoylmethane and Octocrylene in a Microemulsion. *Cosmetics,* **2014**, *1*(2), 128-139.
[http://dx.doi.org/10.3390/cosmetics1020128]

[54] Whitesides, G.M. Nanoscience, nanotechnology, and chemistry. *Small,* **2005**, *1*(2), 172-179.
[http://dx.doi.org/10.1002/smll.200400130] [PMID: 17193427]

[55] Hedberg, J.; Skoglund, S.; Karlsson, M.E.; Wold, S.; Odnevall Wallinder, I.; Hedberg, Y. Sequential studies of silver released from silver nanoparticles in aqueous media simulating sweat, laundry detergent solutions and surface water. *Environ. Sci. Technol.,* **2014**, *48*(13), 7314-7322.
[http://dx.doi.org/10.1021/es500234y] [PMID: 24892700]

[56] Demou, E.; Stark, W.J.; Hellweg, S. Particle emission and exposure during nanoparticle synthesis in research laboratories. *Ann. Occup. Hyg.,* **2009**, *53*(8), 829-838.
[http://dx.doi.org/10.1093/annhyg/mep061] [PMID: 19703918]

[57] Yang, Y.; Colman, B.P.; Bernhardt, E.S.; Hochella, M.F. Importance of a nanoscience approach in the understanding of major aqueous contamination scenarios: case study from a recent coal ash spill. *Environ. Sci. Technol.,* **2015**, *49*(6), 3375-3382.
[http://dx.doi.org/10.1021/es505662q] [PMID: 25688977]

[58] Wiesner, M.R.; Lowry, G.V.; Alvarez, P.; Dionysiou, D.; Biswas, P. Assessing the risks of manufactured nanomaterials. *Environ. Sci. Technol.,* **2006**, *40*(14), 4336-4345.
[http://dx.doi.org/10.1021/es062726m] [PMID: 16903268]

[59] Johnston, L.D.; O'Malley, P.M.; Bachman, J.G. Monitoring the Future: National Results on Adolescent Drug Use: Overview of Key Findings. *Focus Am. Psychiatr. Publ.,* **2003**, *1*(2), 213-234.
[http://dx.doi.org/10.1176/foc.1.2.213]

[60] Firdausy, S.; Mahanani, A.E.E. Legal Protection Effort towards Mark Owner from the Share-in Jar Cosmetic Trade. *SIGn Jurnal Hukum,* **2021**, *3*(1), 26-39.
[http://dx.doi.org/10.37276/sjh.v3i1.113]

[61] Carlson, C.; Hussain, S.M.; Schrand, A.M.; Braydich-Stolle, L.K.; Hess, K.L.; Jones, R.L.; Schlager, J.J. Unique cellular interaction of silver nanoparticles: size-dependent generation of reactive oxygen species. *J. Phys. Chem. B,* **2008**, *112*(43), 13608-13619.
[http://dx.doi.org/10.1021/jp712087m] [PMID: 18831567]

[62] Goodale, A.Y.; Gilmore, M.P.; Griffiths, B.M. 21st-Century Stewardship: Infusing Environmental Stewardship Education with Global Citizenship. *Environ. Educ. Res.,* **2024**, 1-26.
[http://dx.doi.org/10.1080/13504622.2024.2335614]

[63] Guo, Y.; Xu, K.; Wu, C.; Zhao, J.; Xie, Y. Surface chemical-modification for engineering the intrinsic

physical properties of inorganic two-dimensional nanomaterials. *Chem. Soc. Rev.,* **2015**, *44*(3), 637-646.
[http://dx.doi.org/10.1039/C4CS00302K] [PMID: 25406669]

[64]   Trujillo-Reyes, J.; Vilchis-Néstor, A.R.; Majumdar, S.; Peralta-Videa, J.R.; Gardea-Torresdey, J.L. Citric acid modifies surface properties of commercial CeO_2 nanoparticles reducing their toxicity and cerium uptake in radish (*Raphanus sativus*) seedlings. *J. Hazard. Mater.,* **2013**, *263*(Pt 2), 677-684.
[http://dx.doi.org/10.1016/j.jhazmat.2013.10.030] [PMID: 24231324]

[65]   Yokel, R.A.; MacPhail, R.C. Engineered nanomaterials: exposures, hazards, and risk prevention. *J. Occup. Med. Toxicol.,* **2011**, *6*(1), 7.
[http://dx.doi.org/10.1186/1745-6673-6-7] [PMID: 21418643]

[66]   Schulte, P.; Geraci, C.; Zumwalde, R.; Hoover, M.; Castranova, V.; Kuempel, E.; Murashov, V.; Vainio, H.; Savolainen, K. Sharpening the focus on occupational safety and health in nanotechnology. *Scand. J. Work Environ. Health,* **2008**, *34*(6), 471-478.
[http://dx.doi.org/10.5271/sjweh.1292] [PMID: 19137209]

[67]   Trovatti, E.; Fernandes, S.C.M.; Rubatat, L.; Freire, C.S.R.; Silvestre, A.J.D.; Neto, C.P. Sustainable nanocomposite films based on bacterial cellulose and pullulan. *Cellulose,* **2012**, *19*(3), 729-737.
[http://dx.doi.org/10.1007/s10570-012-9673-9]

[68]   Seager, T.P.; Linkov, I. Coupling Multicriteria Decision Analysis and Life Cycle Assessment for Nanomaterials. *J. Ind. Ecol.,* **2008**, *12*(3), 282-285.
[http://dx.doi.org/10.1111/j.1530-9290.2008.00048.x]

[69]   Lowry, G.V.; Gregory, K.B.; Apte, S.C.; Lead, J.R. Transformations of nanomaterials in the environment. *Environ. Sci. Technol.,* **2012**, *46*(13), 6893-6899.
[http://dx.doi.org/10.1021/es300839e] [PMID: 22582927]

[70]   Kuzma, J.; Romanchek, J.; Kokotovich, A. Upstream Oversight Assessment for Agrifood Nanotechnology: A Case Studies Approach. *Risk Analysis,* **2008**.
[http://dx.doi.org/10.1111/j.1539-6924.2008.01071.x]

CHAPTER 9

Ethical and Societal Implications of Nanotechnology

Abstract: Nanotechnology offers immense potential to revolutionize various sectors, from medicine to manufacturing. However, its rapid advancement raises significant ethical and societal challenges. This chapter explores the ethical dilemmas associated with nanotechnology, such as privacy concerns, environmental impact, and media-driven misinformation, highlighting the need to balance innovation with ethical responsibility. Issues of equity and access are also examined, with a focus on disparities in global access to nanotechnology-based solutions and the digital divide, particularly in developing countries. The chapter delves into the transformative effects of nanotechnology on the workforce, discussing potential job displacement, the need for reskilling, and broader societal impacts. Ethical governance and regulation are emphasized, outlining the critical role of governments in oversight, the importance of international cooperation, and the necessity of ethical guidelines for research and development. Public participation in ethical decision-making is also underscored as essential for aligning nanotechnology's development with societal values. This content serves as a comprehensive examination of the complex ethical landscape surrounding nanotechnology and offers insights into how researchers, policymakers, and society can work together to ensure responsible and equitable growth.

Keywords: Ethical, Governance, Guidelines, Misinformation, Public perception, Policies, Regulation, Transformative.

INTRODUCTION

Nanotechnology, the science of manipulating materials on an atomic or molecular scale, is poised to revolutionize a wide range of industries, including medicine, electronics, energy, and materials science. Its applications promise unprecedented advancements, from targeted drug delivery systems that could treat diseases with remarkable precision to lightweight, ultra-strong materials that could change the way we build everything from cars to skyscrapers [1]. However, these groundbreaking possibilities also bring with them profound ethical and societal implications that must be carefully considered. As with any powerful technology, nanotechnology's potential benefits are accompanied by significant risks, and the ethical dilemmas it presents are complex and multifaceted. One of the central ethical concerns with nanotechnology is safety [2]. The ethical concerns associated with nanomedicine revolve around safety, privacy, accessibility, and long-term effects. The potential toxicity of nanoparticles and their unknown long-term impact on human health and the environment raise concerns about patient safety and regulatory oversight. Privacy issues emerge with nano-enabled diagnostic devices that continuously monitor health data, raising questions about data security and consent. Accessibility and equity are also challenges, as advanced nanomedicine treatments may be expensive, potentially widening the gap between different socioeconomic groups. The possibility of unintended genetic or biological modifications raises ethical debates about human enhancement and unforeseen consequences. Addressing these concerns requires clear regulations, thorough clinical testing, and ethical guidelines to ensure the responsible development and application of nanomedicine. Nanoparticles, because of their tiny size, can behave in unpredictable ways in biological systems and the environment. While the ability to engineer materials at the nanoscale offers exciting possibilities, it also raises questions about long-term effects on human health and ecological systems [3]. For instance, nanoparticles used in consumer products, such as cosmetics or sunscreens, may be absorbed by the skin and accumulate in the body, with unknown consequences. Similarly, nanoparticles released into the environment could interact with plants, animals, and microorganisms in unforeseen ways, potentially disrupting ecosystems. The challenge lies in balancing innovation with precaution, ensuring that nanotechnology's development does not outpace our understanding of its risks. Beyond safety concerns, nanotechnology also raises significant ethical questions related to privacy and surveillance. Nanotechnology enables the creation of devices so small they are nearly invisible, which can be used for surveillance or data collection without the knowledge or consent of individuals. This capability could be exploited by governments or corporations, leading to potential violations of privacy and civil liberties. For example, nanosensors embedded in everyday objects could monitor people's behavior and health without their awareness, raising concerns about consent and the right to privacy [4]. These issues necessitate a careful examination of the ethical frameworks that govern the development and use of such technologies, ensuring that their deployment respects individual rights and freedoms. Another critical ethical issue is the potential for nanotechnology to exacerbate social inequalities. Access to cutting-edge nanotechnologies could be limited to wealthy individuals or nations, widening the gap between the rich and the poor [5]. This disparity could manifest in various ways, such as unequal access to advanced medical treatments or clean energy technologies, leading to further social and economic divisions. In developing countries, where resources are already scarce, the introduction of nanotechnology without adequate infrastructure and regulation could result in exploitation or environmental harm. Policymakers must therefore consider how to ensure equitable access to nanotechnology's benefits and prevent its misuse in ways that could harm vulnerable populations.

Nanotechnology's impact on the future of work and society is another area of concern. As nanotechnology integrates into various industries, it could displace jobs, particularly in manufacturing and other labour-intensive sectors [6]. Automation and the development of nano-enhanced materials may reduce the need for human workers, leading to unemployment and social unrest. At the same time, new jobs may emerge in nanotechnology-related fields, but these will likely require specialized skills and education, potentially leaving behind those without access to advanced training [7]. Addressing these challenges will require forward-thinking policies that promote reskilling and education, ensuring that the workforce can adapt to the changes brought about by nanotechnology. The importance of addressing these ethical issues cannot be overstated. Nanotechnology's rapid development and its potential to permeate every aspect of society mean that ethical considerations must be integrated into research and development from the outset [8]. Failure to do so could lead to public mistrust, regulatory backlash, and missed opportunities for innovation. Public perception of nanotechnology will play a crucial role in its adoption and success. Suppose the public perceives nanotechnology as dangerous or ethically questionable in that case, it may face resistance similar to that encountered by other emerging technologies, such as genetically modified organisms (GMOs) or artificial intelligence (AI) [9]. Therefore, transparent communication and public engagement are essential. Researchers, policymakers, and industry leaders must work together to ensure that the public is informed about the benefits and risks of nanotechnology and that ethical concerns are addressed openly and inclusively.

Ethical Dilemmas and Public Perception

Ethical dilemmas in nanotechnology arise from the potential for both tremendous benefits and significant risks associated with its applications. Nanotechnology allows for unprecedented control over materials at the atomic level, leading to innovations that can dramatically improve healthcare, energy efficiency, and environmental protection. However, these advancements also present challenges that are not purely technical but ethical, as discussed in Table **9.1**. For example, the ability to create materials with entirely new properties raises concerns about unforeseen health risks and environmental impacts [10]. The potential for nanomaterials to behave differently than their larger-scale counterparts introduces uncertainty about their long-term safety. Furthermore, the development of nano-enhanced products, such as smart drugs or advanced surveillance technologies, brings up questions about consent, autonomy, and privacy. These ethical dilemmas are complex and multifaceted, requiring careful consideration of how to balance technological progress with respect for human rights and environmental sustainability.

Table 9.1. Case studies of ethical issues in nanotechnology.

Case Study	Ethical Issue	Description	Outcome/Lesson Learned	References
Silver nanoparticles in consumer products	Environmental impact	Widespread use of silver nanoparticles in products like textiles and cosmetics raised concerns about their release into water systems and toxicity to aquatic life.	Regulatory bodies and researchers called for stricter environmental assessments and the development of guidelines for nanoparticle disposal. Increased focus on lifecycle analysis.	[16]
Carbon nanotubes and worker safety	Occupational health and safety	Production of carbon nanotubes posed health risks to workers due to potential inhalation, leading to lung damage similar to asbestos.	Resulted in stricter workplace safety regulations, better personal protective equipment (PPE) standards, and improved risk assessments in manufacturing settings.	[17]
Nano-enabled sunscreens	Public perception and misinformation	Concerns over the safety of nanoparticles in sunscreens, with misinformation spreading about potential skin penetration and toxicity.	Prompted increased public education efforts and transparency from manufacturers, along with more detailed safety testing and labeling requirements	[18]
Nanomedicine and informed consent	Informed consent and patient rights	Experimental nanomedicines in clinical trials raised questions about how much patients understood the risks and benefits of treatments.	Led to the development of clearer, more comprehensive informed consent processes in clinical trials involving nanotechnology-based treatments.	[19]
Nanoelectronics and privacy	Privacy and surveillance	Advances in nanoelectronics, such as nanosensors for surveillance, sparked ethical concerns about privacy infringement and data security.	Sparked debates on the need for privacy laws and the establishment of ethical guidelines for the use of nanotechnology in surveillance and data collection.	[20]

(Table 9.1) cont.....

Case Study	Ethical Issue	Description	Outcome/Lesson Learned	References
Nanotechnology in agriculture	Socioeconomic inequality and global equity	The use of nanotechnology in agriculture, such as nanopesticides, raised concerns about accessibility for small-scale farmers in developing countries.	Highlighted the need for policies ensuring fair access to nanotechnology and support for smallholder farmers to prevent widening socioeconomic disparities.	[21]
Nano-enhanced human implants	Human enhancement and ethical boundaries	Development of nano-enhanced implants, such as brain-computer interfaces, raised ethical issues around human enhancement and the potential for inequality.	Generated discussions on the ethical boundaries of human enhancement, leading to calls for regulations on the use of nanotechnology in augmenting human capabilities.	[22]
Nanomaterials in environmental remediation	Dual-use and ethical responsibility	The use of nanomaterials in environmental cleanup raised concerns about their dual-use potential, such as being repurposed for harmful activities.	Emphasized the need for dual-use governance frameworks and responsible stewardship in the development of nanotechnology for environmental and industrial applications.	[23]
Graphene production and environmental degradation	Environmental justice and sustainability	The extraction and production of graphene, a key nanomaterial, posed significant environmental risks, particularly in resource-rich but regulation-poor regions.	Brought attention to the importance of sustainable practices in nanomaterial production and the need for international regulations to protect vulnerable environments.	[24]
Ethical patenting of nanotechnology innovations	Intellectual property and access to technology	Patent practices in nanotechnology, especially by large corporations, raised concerns about monopolization and access to technology in developing countries.	Highlighted the need for fair patent laws and licensing practices to prevent monopolies and ensure broader access to nanotechnology innovations.	[25]

Public awareness and understanding of nanotechnology play a crucial role in shaping the societal response to this emerging field. Despite its growing presence in consumer products and industrial applications, nanotechnology remains a relatively abstract concept for many people [11]. This lack of understanding can lead to both unrealistic expectations and unfounded fears. For instance, while some may view nanotechnology as a panacea for all technological challenges, others might fear its potential for harm without fully understanding the science behind it. Public education and transparent communication are essential to bridge this knowledge gap [12]. When the public is well-informed, they are more likely to engage in meaningful discussions about the ethical implications of nanotechnology, contributing to a more balanced and informed societal perspective. However, this requires efforts from scientists, educators, and policymakers to make nanotechnology accessible and understandable to a broad audience.

The media plays a critical role in shaping public perception of nanotechnology, but its representation of the field is not always accurate or balanced. Sensationalized reporting can lead to misinformation, where the risks or benefits of nanotechnology are exaggerated, creating either undue fear or unrealistic expectations. For example, the portrayal of nanotechnology in science fiction often focuses on dystopian scenarios, such as "gray goo"—a hypothetical situation where self-replicating nanobots consume all matter on Earth—although such scenarios are scientifically implausible [13]. This type of media representation can contribute to public anxiety and ethical concerns about the loss of control over technology. On the other hand, overly optimistic portrayals may downplay legitimate risks, leading to a lack of critical scrutiny. To address these issues, the media need to provide balanced, fact-based reporting on nanotechnology, highlighting both its potential benefits and the ethical challenges it poses. Additionally, scientists and industry leaders should engage with the media to ensure that accurate information is communicated to the public.

Balancing innovation with ethical considerations is one of the most significant challenges in the development and deployment of nanotechnology. On the one hand, the pursuit of innovation is essential for driving progress and addressing global challenges, such as climate change, disease, and resource scarcity [14]. Nanotechnology has the potential to offer solutions to these pressing issues, but the rush to innovate should not come at the expense of ethical reflection. For example, while nanotechnology can improve drug delivery systems, leading to more effective treatments with fewer side effects, it also raises questions about equity and access—will these advanced treatments be available to all, or only to those who can afford them? Furthermore, the environmental impact of manufacturing and disposing of nanomaterials must be considered, as the introduction of these materials into ecosystems could have unforeseen consequences. Policymakers, researchers, and industry leaders must work together to create a regulatory framework that encourages innovation while ensuring that ethical considerations are not overlooked [15]. This includes conducting thorough risk assessments, promoting transparency in research, and involving the public in decision-making processes. Ethical governance in nanotechnology is not about stifling innovation but about ensuring that it proceeds in a way that is responsible, equitable, and sustainable.

Equity and Access Issues

Disparities in access to nanotechnology-based solutions highlight one of the most significant ethical challenges associated with this emerging field. As nanotechnology advances, it has the potential to revolutionize sectors such as healthcare, energy, and agriculture, offering solutions to some of the world's most pressing problems [26]. However, access to these innovations is not uniformly distributed. Wealthier individuals and countries often have the financial resources, infrastructure, and technical expertise to develop and deploy nanotechnology at a rapid pace, leaving marginalized communities and developing nations behind. This disparity is evident in healthcare, where advanced nanomedicine treatments, such as targeted drug delivery systems or nano-diagnostic tools, may only be available to those who can afford them. The unequal distribution of these technologies risks deepening existing social and economic divides, exacerbating inequalities in health outcomes, education, and quality of life [27]. Addressing these disparities requires a concerted effort to ensure that nanotechnology does not become a luxury available only to a privileged few but rather a tool for global improvement.

Ethical concerns regarding global equity in nanotechnology extend beyond mere access to encompass issues of fairness in research, development, and distribution. The global nature of nanotechnology means that innovations often arise in developed countries, where most research is concentrated [28]. This concentration of knowledge and resources can lead to a form of "technological colonization," where developing countries become dependent on advanced economies for access to cutting-edge technologies. Furthermore, the benefits of nanotechnology are often unevenly distributed, with wealthier nations reaping the rewards while poorer nations bear the risks, such as environmental degradation or exploitation of natural resources. For example, developing countries might be used as testing grounds for new nanotechnologies or as sources of raw materials, without receiving a fair share of the benefits [29]. These ethical concerns demand a reevaluation of global partnerships in nanotechnology, ensuring that collaboration is based on mutual benefit, respect, and equitable sharing of knowledge and resources.

The impact of nanotechnology on developing countries is a double-edged sword. On one hand, nanotechnology offers immense potential to address challenges that disproportionately affect these regions, such as water purification, agricultural productivity, and disease management. For example, inexpensive nanofilters could provide clean drinking water, and nano-fertilizers could enhance crop yields in resource-poor settings [30]. On the other hand, the introduction of nanotechnology into developing countries without proper infrastructure and regulation could lead to exploitation and harm. Developing countries may lack the capacity to assess the safety and environmental impact of nanomaterials, leading to health risks and ecological damage. Additionally, the influx of nanotechnology-based products from developed countries could displace local industries and exacerbate economic inequalities. To ensure that nanotechnology benefits rather than harms developing nations, it is crucial to establish frameworks that promote capacity-building, technology transfer, and ethical business practices [31]. This includes providing training and resources to enable developing countries to participate in the global nanotechnology economy on an equal footing.

The digital divide, which refers to the gap between those who have access to digital technologies and those who do not, is closely linked to issues of equity and access in nanotechnology. As nanotechnology increasingly intersects with information technology, the digital divide threatens to widen. Advanced nanotechnologies often rely on digital infrastructure for their development, deployment, and use—whether it be in the form of data analytics, machine learning, or internet connectivity [32]. In regions where access to digital technology is limited, the benefits of nanotechnology may remain out of reach. For example, rural areas without reliable internet access may not be able to utilize nano-enabled agricultural sensors or health monitoring devices that depend on connectivity [33]. This digital divide exacerbates existing inequalities, as those without access to digital technologies are also excluded from the opportunities that nanotechnology offers. Bridging this divide is essential for ensuring that nanotechnology serves as a tool for global equity rather than a driver of further inequality.

Addressing equity and access issues in nanotechnology requires robust and inclusive policy frameworks at both national and international levels, as depicted in Fig. (**9.1**). Policymakers must prioritize the development of regulations that ensure fair distribution of nanotechnology's benefits while minimizing its risks. This includes promoting equitable access to nanotechnology-based healthcare, education, and infrastructure, particularly in underserved communities and developing countries [34]. International collaboration is key to achieving these goals, with developed countries playing a supportive role in technology transfer and capacity-building initiatives [35]. Additionally, policies should encourage responsible innovation that considers the social and environmental impacts of nanotechnology from the outset. Public funding for nanotechnology research should be directed not only toward cutting-edge innovations but also toward applications that address the needs of disadvantaged populations, such as affordable healthcare solutions and sustainable agricultural practices. Furthermore, ethical guidelines must be established to prevent exploitation and ensure that all stakeholders, including marginalized communities, have a voice in decision-making processes. By implementing these policy recommendations, we can work towards a future where nanotechnology contributes to a more equitable and just world.

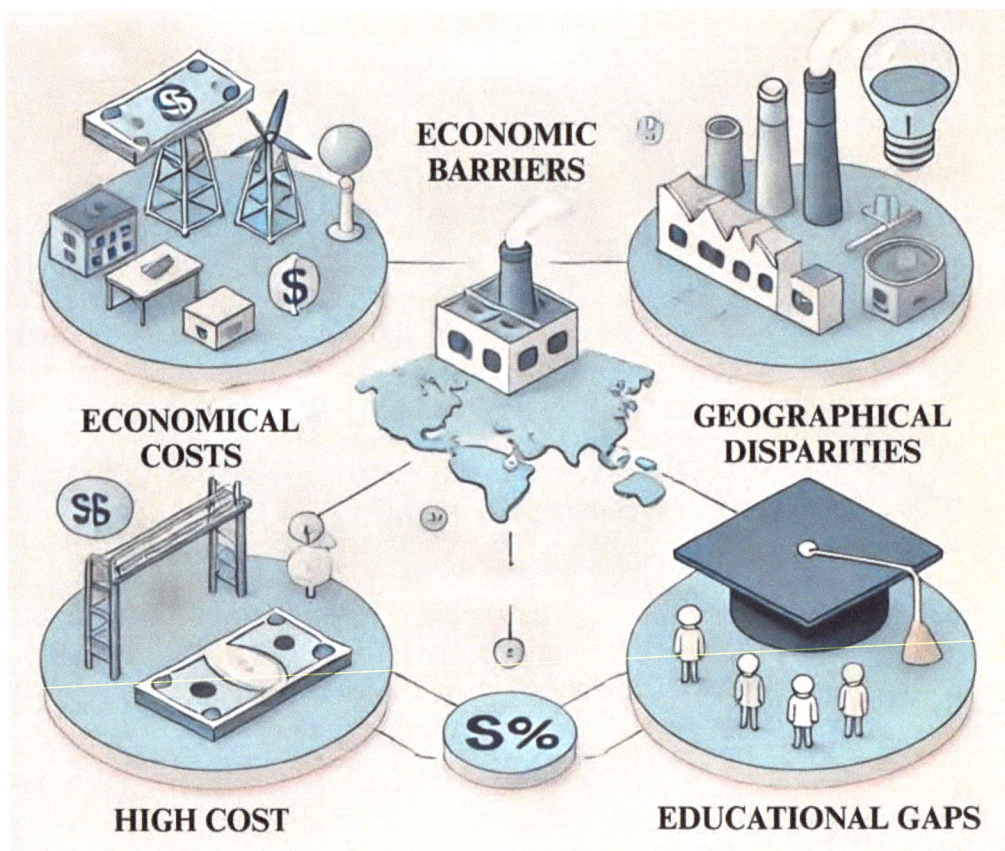

Fig. (9.1). Equity and access issues in nanotechnology.

THE FUTURE OF WORK AND SOCIETY WITH NANOTECHNOLOGY

Nanotechnology is poised to be a major force in transforming the employment landscape across various industries. As nanotechnology continues to advance, it will lead to the creation of new jobs and industries that did not exist before, such as in the fields of nano-manufacturing, nano-medicine, and nanoelectronics.

These new opportunities will require a workforce with specialized skills in nanoscience, engineering, and technology, driving demand for education and training in these areas. Industries like healthcare, electronics, energy, and materials science will particularly benefit from the innovations brought by nanotechnology, leading to the emergence of roles that focus on the design, development, and maintenance of nano-enabled products and systems [36]. However, this transformative potential also brings challenges. Traditional manufacturing jobs, especially those in industries that rely heavily on materials processing and assembly, may face disruption as nanotechnology enables more efficient, automated processes. Workers in these sectors may find themselves needing to adapt to new technologies or face the risk of job displacement. The overall impact of nanotechnology on employment will be significant, reshaping the job market and requiring a proactive approach to workforce development to ensure that workers are prepared for the changes ahead.

One of the most pressing concerns associated with the rise of nanotechnology is the potential for job displacement. As nanotechnology enhances automation and enables more efficient manufacturing processes, jobs that once required human labor may become obsolete [37]. For instance, the development of nano-robots capable of performing complex tasks with precision could reduce the need for certain skilled labor in fields like surgery, manufacturing, and even environmental monitoring [38]. This displacement poses a significant challenge to the workforce, particularly for workers who lack the skills or resources to transition into new roles. To mitigate the impact of job displacement, there will be a critical need for reskilling and upskilling programs. Governments, educational institutions, and industries must collaborate to develop training initiatives that equip workers with the necessary skills to thrive in a nanotechnology-driven economy [39]. This could include retraining programs focused on advanced manufacturing techniques, nanomaterials science, or other emerging fields. Furthermore, there should be a focus on fostering adaptability and lifelong learning among workers, enabling them to continuously upgrade their skills in response to technological advancements. Addressing the reskilling needs of the workforce will be essential to ensure that the benefits of nanotechnology are shared broadly and that workers are not left behind in the transition.

The adoption of nanotechnology will have far-reaching social impacts, influencing various aspects of daily life, economic structures, and societal norms. Nanotechnology has the potential to improve quality of life by offering breakthroughs in healthcare, environmental protection, and energy efficiency. For example, advancements in nano-medicine could lead to more effective treatments for chronic diseases, while nano-enabled environmental technologies could help address pollution and climate change [40]. However, the widespread adoption of nanotechnology also raises concerns about social inequality. If access to nanotechnology-based products and services is not equitably distributed, it could exacerbate existing social divides, creating a gap between those who can afford the latest technological innovations and those who cannot. Additionally, the integration of nanotechnology into everyday products may raise privacy and security concerns, particularly with the use of nanosensors and other monitoring technologies. As nanotechnology becomes more embedded in society, it will be crucial to consider its social implications and to develop policies that promote inclusivity, protect privacy, and ensure that the benefits of nanotechnology are accessible to all segments of society.

The workforce transformation driven by nanotechnology presents several ethical challenges that must be carefully navigated. One of the primary concerns is the potential for increased economic inequality. As high-paying jobs in nanotechnology-related fields proliferate, there is a risk that workers without access to the necessary education and training may be left behind, leading to a widening income gap. This scenario raises questions about fairness and justice in the distribution of technological benefits [41]. Additionally, the shift towards automation and the use of nano-robots in various industries could lead to job losses, particularly in sectors that have traditionally provided stable employment for low- and middle-skilled workers. The ethical challenge lies in balancing the pursuit of technological progress with the need to protect workers' rights and livelihoods. Employers, policymakers, and society at large must consider how to support displaced workers, whether through reskilling programs, social safety nets, or new forms of employment that leverage human skills alongside technological advancements. There is an ethical imperative to ensure that the transition to a nanotechnology-driven economy does not disproportionately impact vulnerable populations, such as those in rural areas or developing countries, who may lack access to the resources needed to adapt to these changes.

The long-term societal implications of nanotechnology are profound, touching on issues of sustainability, economic stability, and social cohesion. In the long run, nanotechnology has the potential to contribute significantly to sustainable development by enabling the creation of more efficient energy systems, reducing waste through advanced materials, and mitigating environmental damage through innovative clean-up technologies. However, these benefits must be weighed against the potential risks, such as the environmental and health impacts of nanomaterials, which are not yet fully understood [42]. The sustainability of nanotechnology will depend on the development of robust regulatory frameworks that ensure the safe use of nanomaterials, as well as ongoing research into their long-term effects. Additionally, the societal implications of nanotechnology extend to the ethical considerations of its use in areas like human enhancement, where the line between therapeutic and enhancement applications may blur, raising questions about equity, consent, and the definition of what it means to be human [43]. As nanotechnology continues to evolve, it will be essential to engage in ongoing dialogue about its societal impacts, involving diverse stakeholders, including scientists, ethicists, policymakers, and the public. This dialogue should aim to anticipate and address the challenges that nanotechnology poses to society, ensuring that its development is guided by principles of sustainability, equity, and social responsibility.

ETHICAL GOVERNANCE AND REGULATION

Governments play a crucial role in providing ethical oversight for the development and application of nanotechnology [44]. As the field rapidly evolves, national governments must establish robust regulatory frameworks to ensure that nanotechnology is developed responsibly and safely. This oversight involves creating regulations that address the unique challenges posed by nanomaterials, such as their potential environmental and health impacts, and ensuring that these regulations are regularly updated as new scientific data emerges. Governments must also balance the promotion of innovation with the protection of public interests, avoiding overly restrictive regulations that could stifle technological progress while preventing harm to society. Moreover, governments need to consider ethical issues such as privacy, consent, and equity, particularly in areas like healthcare and surveillance, where nanotechnology can have profound societal impacts. By setting clear ethical guidelines and enforcing compliance, governments can help ensure that nanotechnology is developed in a way that aligns with societal values and protects public welfare.

Nanotechnology's global nature necessitates international cooperation and harmonization of regulations. Given the cross-border implications of nanomaterial production, usage, and disposal, countries must collaborate to create consistent standards that ensure safety and ethical conduct worldwide [45]. International organizations such as the United Nations, the World Health Organization, and the Organisation for Economic Co-operation and Development (OECD) play a pivotal role in facilitating this cooperation by providing platforms for dialogue and consensus-building among nations [46]. These organizations can help develop international treaties and agreements that address key issues such as environmental sustainability, labour rights, and fair-trade practices related to nanotechnology. In addition, global cooperation is vital for addressing ethical concerns related to nanotechnology in areas like biomedicine and artificial intelligence, where different cultural perspectives and values may influence regulatory approaches [47]. By fostering international collaboration and creating shared frameworks, the global community can work towards ensuring that nanotechnology is developed ethically and safely across borders, while also promoting equitable access to its benefits.

The establishment of ethical guidelines for nanotechnology research and development (R&D) is essential to ensure that scientific advancements align with societal values and do not compromise ethical principles. These guidelines should cover a wide range of issues, including the safety of research subjects, the responsible use of resources, and the transparency of research processes [48]. For instance, ethical guidelines can help prevent potential harm to human participants in clinical trials involving nanomedicine by requiring thorough risk assessments and informed consent procedures. In addition, guidelines should address the environmental implications of nanotechnology research, ensuring that experiments involving nanomaterials are conducted in a way that minimizes ecological impact. Researchers and developers must also consider the broader societal implications of their work, such as the potential for nanotechnology to exacerbate social inequalities or contribute to unethical practices like surveillance or human enhancement. To be effective, these guidelines should be developed collaboratively by scientists, ethicists, policymakers, and other stakeholders, and should be enforced by both national and international regulatory bodies [49]. By adhering to ethical guidelines, the scientific community can ensure that nanotechnology R&D proceeds in a manner that respects human dignity, protects the environment, and promotes social good.

Public participation is a key component of ethical governance in nanotechnology, as it ensures that the development and regulation of this technology reflect the values and concerns of society at large [50]. Engaging the public in ethical decision-making can help bridge the gap between scientific innovation and societal expectations, fostering greater transparency, trust, and accountability in the process. This participation can take many forms, including public consultations, citizen panels, and participatory technology assessments, where diverse groups of people are invited to discuss and provide input on nanotechnology-related issues. By involving the public in discussions about the risks and benefits of nanotechnology, policymakers can better understand the ethical concerns of different communities and make more informed decisions that take into account diverse perspectives. Public participation also serves to democratize the governance of nanotechnology, ensuring that decisions are not solely driven by industry interests or scientific elites, but are instead grounded in the collective wisdom of society [51]. Educating the public about nanotechnology and its ethical implications is crucial for enabling meaningful participation. This requires efforts to improve science literacy and provide accessible information about the technology's potential impacts. Ultimately, public participation in ethical decision-making can help ensure that nanotechnology is developed in a way that is socially responsible, ethically sound, and aligned with the values of the broader community [52]. Some of the challenges that are associated with the regulation of nanotechnology are depicted in Fig. (**9.2**).

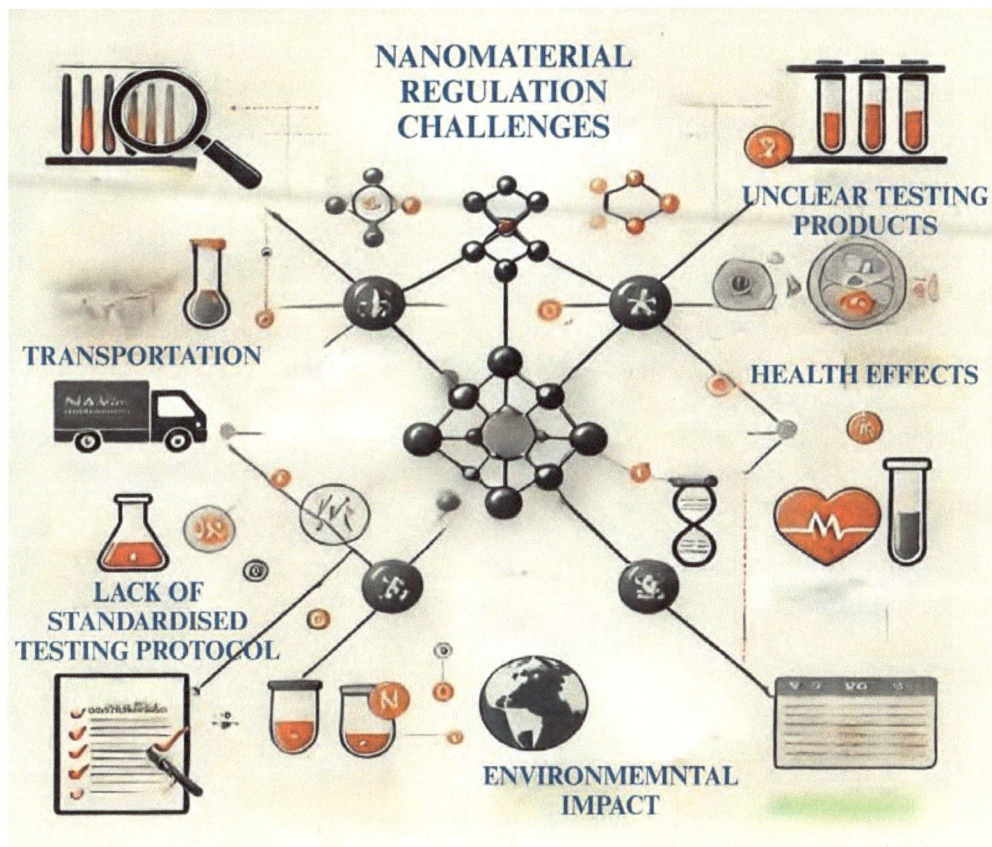

Fig. (**9.2**). Nanomaterials regulation challenges.

CONCLUSION

Nanotechnology, with its transformative potential across various sectors, brings to the forefront several key ethical and societal issues. These include ethical dilemmas related to privacy, safety, and environmental impact; disparities in access to nanotechnology-based solutions; and concerns about its effects on employment and society. As the technology advances, it raises questions about how to balance innovation with ethical responsibility, ensuring that the benefits of nanotechnology are distributed equitably across society while minimizing risks. Global equity and the digital divide further complicate these issues, particularly for developing countries that may be left behind in the nanotechnology revolution. Additionally, the societal impacts of workforce transformation and the potential for job displacement highlight the need for careful consideration of the long-term implications of widespread nanotechnology adoption. The regulatory landscape must also evolve to address these concerns, requiring a coordinated effort between governments, international bodies, and public stakeholders.

The path forward requires a delicate balance between fostering technological progress and upholding ethical principles. As nanotechnology continues to evolve, researchers, policymakers, and industry leaders must work together to create frameworks that prioritize safety, equity, and sustainability. Ethical governance must be proactive rather than reactive, anticipating potential risks and addressing them before they become widespread. This involves establishing clear ethical guidelines for research and development, ensuring that regulations keep pace with innovation, and promoting international cooperation to harmonize standards across borders. Equally important is the need to address societal concerns, such as job displacement and access to technology, by implementing policies that support reskilling, education, and equitable distribution of nanotechnology's benefits. By taking a holistic approach that integrates ethical considerations into every stage of nanotechnology's development, society can ensure that the technology serves the greater good without compromising its values.

The responsibility for ensuring the ethical and equitable development of nanotechnology does not rest on one group alone; it requires a collective effort from researchers, policymakers, and society at large. Researchers must prioritize ethical considerations in their work, conducting studies with transparency and a commitment to minimizing harm. Policymakers need to establish and enforce regulations that protect public welfare while encouraging innovation. They must also engage with international partners to create consistent global standards. Society, on the other hand, must stay informed and participate in the dialogue surrounding nanotechnology, ensuring that their voices are heard in decision-making processes. Public participation in ethical discussions is vital to ensuring that nanotechnology's development reflects the values and concerns of the broader community. Together, these stakeholders can help navigate the ethical challenges of nanotechnology, ensuring that its benefits are realized in a way that is just, sustainable, and aligned with societal values. This collective action will be critical in shaping a future where nanotechnology contributes to human progress while respecting ethical boundaries.

REFERENCES

[1]   Tomalia, D.A. Birth of a new macromolecular architecture: dendrimers as quantized building blocks for nanoscale synthetic polymer chemistry. *Prog. Polym. Sci.,* **2005**, *30*(3-4), 294-324. [http://dx.doi.org/10.1016/j.progpolymsci.2005.01.007]

[2]   Anand, M.; Srivastava, N.; Sarma, S. Policy and ethical concerns in nanotechnology safety: case of Indian health sector. *J. Biomed. Nanotechnol.,* **2011**, *7*(1), 34-35.

[http://dx.doi.org/10.1166/jbn.2011.1188] [PMID: 21485790]

[3]   Dong, A.; Ye, X.; Chen, J.; Kang, Y.; Gordon, T.; Kikkawa, J.M.; Murray, C.B. A generalized ligand-exchange strategy enabling sequential surface functionalization of colloidal nanocrystals. *J. Am. Chem. Soc.,* **2011**, *133*(4), 998-1006.
[http://dx.doi.org/10.1021/ja108948z] [PMID: 21175183]

[4]   Kuznetsov, D.; Dezhurov, S.; Krylsky, D.; Neschisliaev, V. Fluorescent nanosensors for molecular visualization of the c-Met tumor marker. *Nano-Structures & Nano-Objects,* **2022**, *31*, 100890.
[http://dx.doi.org/10.1016/j.nanoso.2022.100890]

[5]   Nel, A.E.; Mädler, L.; Velegol, D.; Xia, T.; Hoek, E.M.V.; Somasundaran, P.; Klaessig, F.; Castranova, V.; Thompson, M. Understanding biophysicochemical interactions at the nano–bio interface. *Nat. Mater.,* **2009**, *8*(7), 543-557.
[http://dx.doi.org/10.1038/nmat2442] [PMID: 19525947]

[6]   Baughman, R.H.; Zakhidov, A.A.; de Heer, W.A. Carbon nanotubes--the route toward applications. *Science,* **2002**, *297*(5582), 787-792.
[http://dx.doi.org/10.1126/science.1060928] [PMID: 12161643]

[7]   Roco, M.C. The long view of nanotechnology development: the National Nanotechnology Initiative at 10 years. *J. Nanopart. Res.,* **2011**, *13*(2), 427-445.
[http://dx.doi.org/10.1007/s11051-010-0192-z]

[8]   Lopez, A.P. Nanomedicine and its Potential in Managing Diabetes. *Nanotechnology and Nanomaterials Research,* **2020**, *1*(1).
[http://dx.doi.org/10.47275/2692-885X-102]

[9]   Sylvester, D.J.; Abbott, K.W.; Marchant, G.E. Not again! Public perception, regulation, and nanotechnology. *Regul. Gov.,* **2009**, *3*(2), 165-185.
[http://dx.doi.org/10.1111/j.1748-5991.2009.01049.x]

[10]   Sealy, C. Chimeric proteins create new nanocomposite. *Mater. Today,* **2006**, *9*(7-8), 18.
[http://dx.doi.org/10.1016/S1369-7021(06)71571-1]

[11]   Whitesides, G.M.; Boncheva, M. Beyond molecules: Self-assembly of mesoscopic and macroscopic components. *Proc. Natl. Acad. Sci. USA,* **2002**, *99*(8), 4769-4774.
[http://dx.doi.org/10.1073/pnas.082065899] [PMID: 11959929]

[12]   Alvarez, P.J.J.; Chan, C.K.; Elimelech, M.; Halas, N.J.; Villagrán, D. Emerging opportunities for nanotechnology to enhance water security. *Nat. Nanotechnol.,* **2018**, *13*(8), 634-641.
[http://dx.doi.org/10.1038/s41565-018-0203-2] [PMID: 30082804]

[13]   Vitaliev, V. After all...of foglets and nanobots. *Engineering & Technology,* **2007**, *2*(8), 64-64.
[http://dx.doi.org/10.1049/et:20070816]

[14]   Arora, A.; Arora, A. Generative adversarial networks and synthetic patient data: current challenges and future perspectives. *Future Healthc. J.,* **2022**, *9*(2), 190-193.
[http://dx.doi.org/10.7861/fhj.2022-0013] [PMID: 35928184]

[15]   Sheldon, R.A. Metrics of Green Chemistry and Sustainability: Past, Present, and Future. *ACS Sustain. Chem.& Eng.,* **2018**, *6*(1), 32-48.
[http://dx.doi.org/10.1021/acssuschemeng.7b03505]

[16]   Quadros, M.E.; Marr, L.C. Silver nanoparticles and total aerosols emitted by nanotechnology-related consumer spray products. *Environ. Sci. Technol.,* **2011**, *45*(24), 10713-10719.
[http://dx.doi.org/10.1021/es202770m] [PMID: 22070550]

[17]   Aricò, A.S.; Bruce, P.; Scrosati, B.; Tarascon, J.M.; van Schalkwijk, W. Nanostructured materials for advanced energy conversion and storage devices. *Nat. Mater.,* **2005**, *4*(5), 366-377.
[http://dx.doi.org/10.1038/nmat1368] [PMID: 15867920]

[18]   Kessler, R. Engineered nanoparticles in consumer products: understanding a new ingredient. *Environ.*

Health Perspect., **2011**, *119*(3), a120-a125.
[http://dx.doi.org/10.1289/ehp.119-a120] [PMID: 21356630]

[19]   King, N.M.P. Nanomedicine first-in-human research: challenges for informed consent. *J. Law Med. Ethics,* **2012**, *40*(4), 823-830.
[http://dx.doi.org/10.1111/j.1748-720X.2012.00710.x] [PMID: 23289684]

[20]   Balandin, A.A. *Journal of Nanoelectronics and Optoelectronics:* Entering the Third Year. *Journal of Nanoelectronics and Optoelectronics,* **2008**, *3*(1), 1-1.
[http://dx.doi.org/10.1166/jno.2008.001]

[21]   B, S. Nanotechnology in Agriculture. *J. Nanomed. Nanotechnol.,* **2011**, *2*(7).
[http://dx.doi.org/10.4172/2157-7439.1000123]

[22]   Bhadra, C.M.; Khanh Truong, V.; Pham, V.T.H.; Al Kobaisi, M.; Seniutinas, G.; Wang, J.Y.; Juodkazis, S.; Crawford, R.J.; Ivanova, E.P. Antibacterial titanium nano-patterned arrays inspired by dragonfly wings. *Sci. Rep.,* **2015**, *5*(1), 16817.
[http://dx.doi.org/10.1038/srep16817] [PMID: 26576662]

[23]   Khin, M.M.; Nair, A.S.; Babu, V.J.; Murugan, R.; Ramakrishna, S. A review on nanomaterials for environmental remediation. *Energy Environ. Sci.,* **2012**, *5*(8), 8075.
[http://dx.doi.org/10.1039/c2ee21818f]

[24]   Han, L.; Wang, P.; Dong, S. Progress in graphene-based photoactive nanocomposites as a promising class of photocatalyst. *Nanoscale,* **2012**, *4*(19), 5814-5825.
[http://dx.doi.org/10.1039/c2nr31699d] [PMID: 22910810]

[25]   Nanotechnology: Science, Innovation and Opportunity. *Choice Reviews Online,* **2006**, *44*(1), 027144-0271.
[http://dx.doi.org/10.5860/CHOICE.44-0271]

[26]   Tan, C.; Cao, X.; Wu, X.J.; He, Q.; Yang, J.; Zhang, X.; Chen, J.; Zhao, W.; Han, S.; Nam, G.H.; Sindoro, M.; Zhang, H. Recent Advances in Ultrathin Two-Dimensional Nanomaterials. *Chem. Rev.,* **2017**, *117*(9), 6225-6331.
[http://dx.doi.org/10.1021/acs.chemrev.6b00558] [PMID: 28306244]

[27]   Mensah, J. Sustainable development: Meaning, history, principles, pillars, and implications for human action: Literature review. *Cogent Soc. Sci.,* **2019**, *5*(1), 1653531.
[http://dx.doi.org/10.1080/23311886.2019.1653531]

[28]   Pendergast, M.M.; Hoek, E.M.V. A review of water treatment membrane nanotechnologies. *Energy Environ. Sci.,* **2011**, *4*(6), 1946.
[http://dx.doi.org/10.1039/c0ee00541j]

[29]   Hauck, T.S.; Giri, S.; Gao, Y.; Chan, W.C.W. Nanotechnology diagnostics for infectious diseases prevalent in developing countries. *Adv. Drug Deliv. Rev.,* **2010**, *62*(4-5), 438-448.
[http://dx.doi.org/10.1016/j.addr.2009.11.015] [PMID: 19931580]

[30]   Botes, M.; Eugene Cloete, T. The potential of nanofibers and nanobiocides in water purification. *Crit. Rev. Microbiol.,* **2010**, *36*(1), 68-81.
[http://dx.doi.org/10.3109/10408410903397332] [PMID: 20088684]

[31]   The Road to Green Nanotechnology *J. Ind. Ecol.,* **2008**, *12*(3), 263-266.
[http://dx.doi.org/10.1111/j.1530-9290.2008.00045.x]

[32]   Sharma, S.; Alam, M.A.; Sharma, A.; Singh, P.; Dhoundiyal, S.; Sharma, A. High-Impact Applications of IoT System-Based Metaheuristics. In: *Nature-Inspired Methods for Smart Healthcare Systems and Medical Data*; Springer Nature: Switzerland, **2023**; pp. 121-131.

[33]   Xin, X.; Judy, J.D.; Sumerlin, B.B.; He, Z. Nano-enabled agriculture: from nanoparticles to smart nanodelivery systems. *Environ. Chem.,* **2020**, *17*(6), 413.
[http://dx.doi.org/10.1071/EN19254]

[34]   Colvin, V.L. The potential environmental impact of engineered nanomaterials. *Nat. Biotechnol.,* **2003**, *21*(10), 1166-1170.
[http://dx.doi.org/10.1038/nbt875] [PMID: 14520401]

[35]   Zheng, J.; Zhao, Z.; Zhang, X.; Chen, D.; Huang, M. International collaboration development in nanotechnology: a perspective of patent network analysis. *Scientometrics,* **2014**, *98*(1), 683-702.
[http://dx.doi.org/10.1007/s11192-013-1081-x]

[36]   Zeng, W.; Shu, L.; Li, Q.; Chen, S.; Wang, F.; Tao, X.M. Fiber-based wearable electronics: a review of materials, fabrication, devices, and applications. *Adv. Mater.,* **2014**, *26*(31), 5310-5336.
[http://dx.doi.org/10.1002/adma.201400633] [PMID: 24943999]

[37]   Qu, X.; Alvarez, P.J.J.; Li, Q. Applications of nanotechnology in water and wastewater treatment. *Water Res.,* **2013**, *47*(12), 3931-3946.
[http://dx.doi.org/10.1016/j.watres.2012.09.058] [PMID: 23571110]

[38]   Li, J.; Esteban-Fernández de Ávila, B.; Gao, W.; Zhang, L.; Wang, J. Micro/nanorobots for biomedicine: Delivery, surgery, sensing, and detoxification. *Sci. Robot.,* **2017**, *2*(4).
[http://dx.doi.org/10.1126/scirobotics.aam6431] [PMID: 31552379]

[39]   Schot, J.; Steinmueller, W.E. Three frames for innovation policy: R&D, systems of innovation and transformative change. *Res. Policy,* **2018**, *47*(9), 1554-1567.
[http://dx.doi.org/10.1016/j.respol.2018.08.011]

[40]   Nanopillars, C.S.C.; More Efficient, S.C. Nanopillars could spell cheaper, more efficient solar cells. *Nano Today,* **2009**, *4*(5), 379.
[http://dx.doi.org/10.1016/j.nantod.2009.08.004]

[41]   Roco, M.C. The long view of nanotechnology development: the National Nanotechnology Initiative at 10 years. *J. Nanopart. Res.,* **2011**, *13*(2), 427-445.
[http://dx.doi.org/10.1007/s11051-010-0192-z]

[42]   Lillian, S. *Nanotechnology Research Increases Significantly*; Nature Africa, **2021**.
[http://dx.doi.org/10.1038/d44148-021-00069-2]

[43]   Nanotechnology: Societal Implications. *Nano Today,* **2006**, *1*(4), 41.
[http://dx.doi.org/10.1016/S1748-0132(06)70121-9]

[44]   Ramachandraiah, K.; Han, S.G.; Chin, K.B. Nanotechnology in meat processing and packaging: potential applications - a review. *Asian-Australas. J. Anim. Sci.,* **2015**, *28*(2), 290-302.
[http://dx.doi.org/10.5713/ajas.14.0607] [PMID: 25557827]

[45]   Peters, R.; Brandhoff, P.; Weigel, S.; Marvin, H.; Bouwmeester, H.; Aschberger, K.; Rauscher, H.; Amenta, V.; Arena, M.; Botelho Moniz, F.; Gottardo, S.; Mech, A. Inventory of Nanotechnology applications in the agricultural, feed and food sector. *EFSA Support. Publ.,* **2014**, *11*(7).
[http://dx.doi.org/10.2903/sp.efsa.2014.EN-621]

[46]   Mbengue, M.M.; Charles, M. International Organizations and Nanotechnologies: The Challenge of Coordination. *Rev. Eur. Comp. Int. Environ. Law,* **2013**, *22*(2), 174-185.
[http://dx.doi.org/10.1111/reel.12033]

[47]   Moor, J.; Weckert, J. Nanoethics: Assessing the Nanoscale from an Ethical Point of View. 2004, 301–310.

[48]   Duncan, T.V. Applications of nanotechnology in food packaging and food safety: Barrier materials, antimicrobials and sensors. *J. Colloid Interface Sci.,* **2011**, *363*(1), 1-24.
[http://dx.doi.org/10.1016/j.jcis.2011.07.017] [PMID: 21824625]

[49]   Powell, M.; Lee Kleinman, D. Building citizen capacities for participation in nanotechnology decision-making: the democratic virtues of the consensus Conference model. *Public Underst. Sci.,* **2008**, *17*(3), 329-348.
[http://dx.doi.org/10.1177/0963662506068000]

[50] Sandoval, B.M. Perspectives on FDA's Regulation of Nanotechnology: Emerging Challenges and Potential Solutions. *Compr. Rev. Food Sci. Food Saf.,* **2009**, *8*(4), 375-393.
[http://dx.doi.org/10.1111/j.1541-4337.2009.00088.x]

[51] L Feitshans, I. Nanotechnology Revolutionizing Public Health for the Covid-19 Era. *Nanomedicine & Nanotechnology Open Access,* **2020**, *5*(3).
[http://dx.doi.org/10.23880/NNOA-16000192]

[52] Lee, M. Risk and Beyond: EU Regulation of Nanotechnology. *Eur. Law Rev.,* **2010**, (6), 799-821.

SUBJECT INDEX

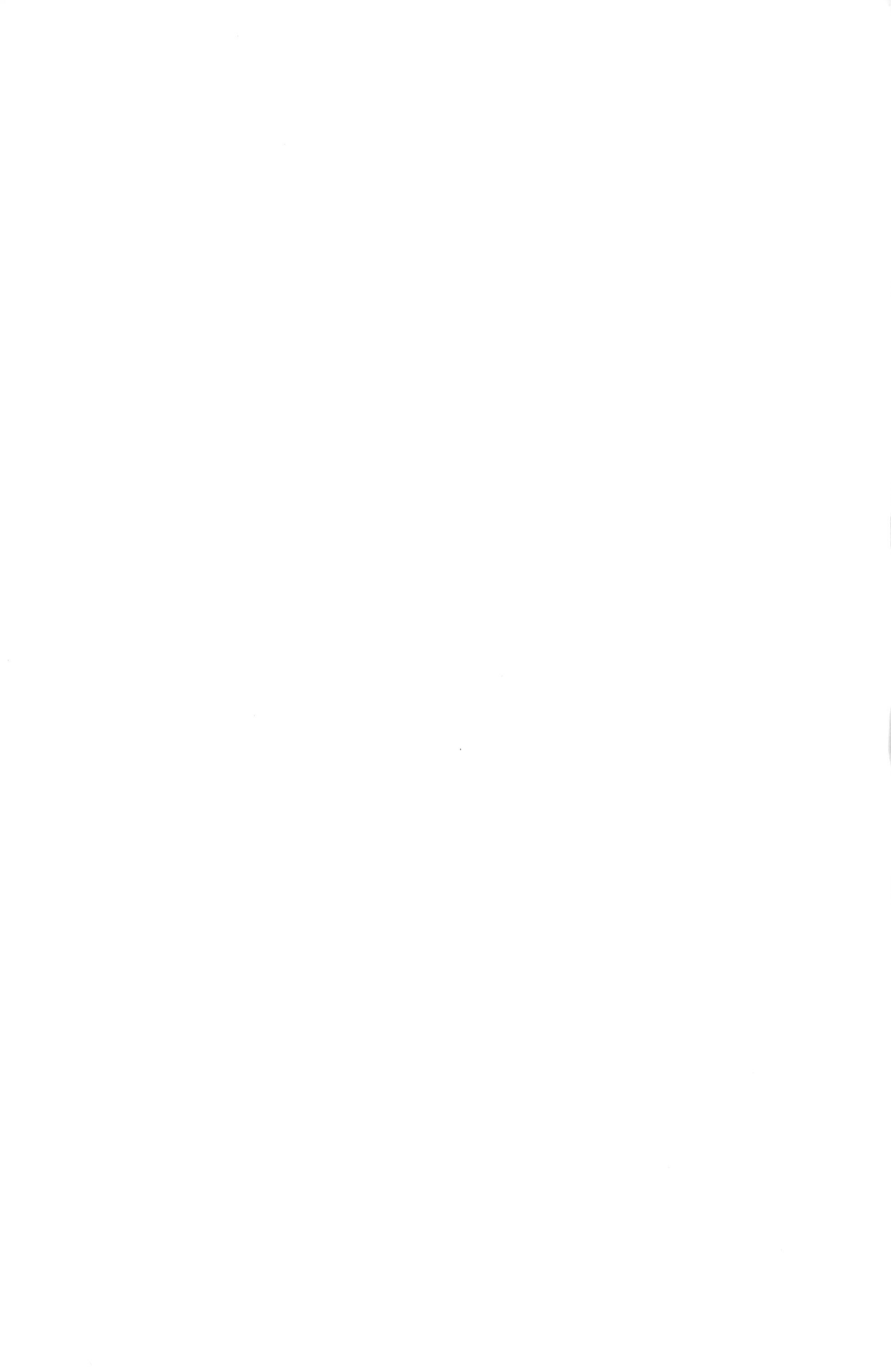

www.ingramcontent.com/pod-product-compliance
Lightning Source LLC
Chambersburg PA
CBHW041658210326
41598CB00007B/454